# Oops, I Packed My Trauma

*A Fun and Transformative Guide to Energy Healing*

Emmy Violet

© **Copyright 2024 - All rights reserved.**

The content contained within this book may not be reproduced, duplicated or transmitted without direct written permission from the author or the publisher.

Under no circumstances will any blame or legal responsibility be held against the publisher, or author, for any damages, reparation, or monetary loss due to the information contained within this book, either directly or indirectly.

Legal Notice:

This book is copyright protected. It is only for personal use. You cannot amend, distribute, sell, use, quote or paraphrase any part, or the content within this book, without the consent of the author or publisher.

Disclaimer Notice:

Please note the information contained within this document is for educational and entertainment purposes only. All effort has been executed to present accurate, up to date, reliable, complete information. No warranties of any kind are declared or implied. Readers acknowledge that the author is not engaged in the rendering of legal, financial, medical or professional advice. The content within this book has been derived from various sources. Please consult a licensed professional before attempting any techniques outlined in this book.

By reading this document, the reader agrees that under no circumstances is the author responsible for any losses, direct or indirect, that are incurred as a result of the use of the information contained within this document, including, but not limited to, errors, omissions, or inaccuracies.

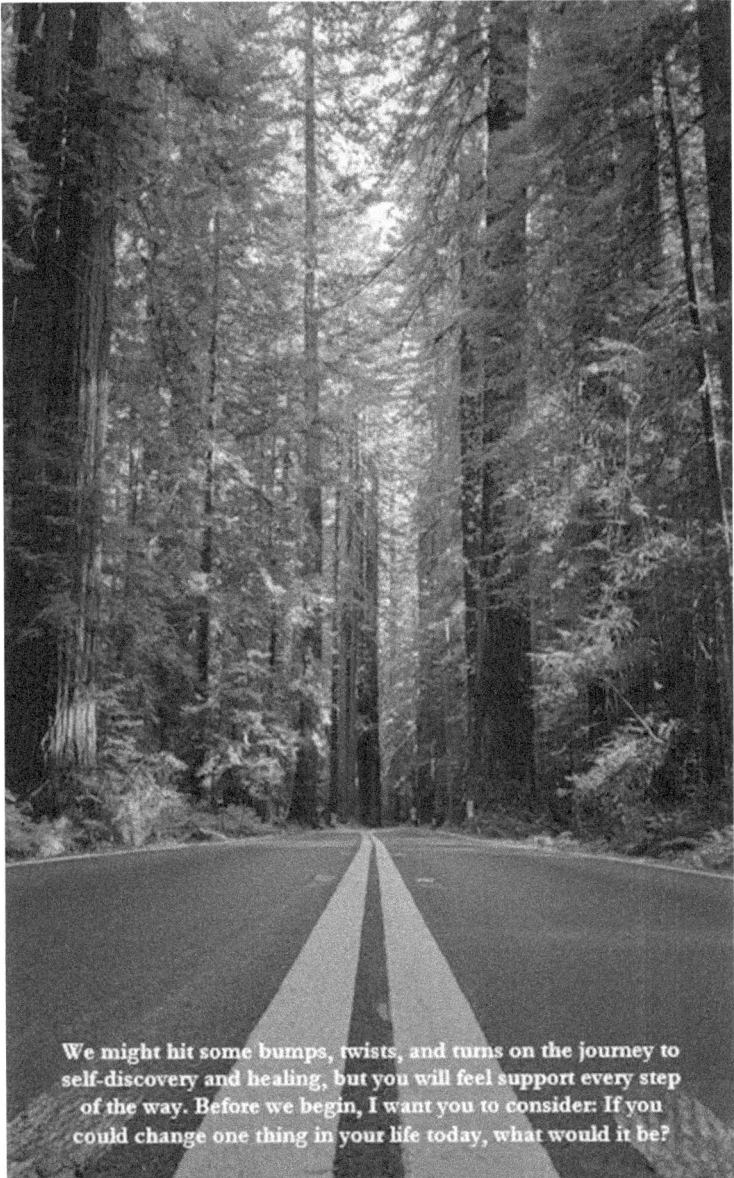

We might hit some bumps, twists, and turns on the journey to self-discovery and healing, but you will feel support every step of the way. Before we begin, I want you to consider: If you could change one thing in your life today, what would it be?

# Table of Contents

**ABOUT THE AUTHOR** ..................................................................1

**INTRODUCTION** ........................................................................3

**CHAPTER 1: THE MIND-BODY CONNECTION** ...........................7
   UNDERSTANDING THE BODY'S ENERGY SYSTEM ................................... 7
   THE LINK BETWEEN MIND, BODY, AND ENERGY SYSTEM ....................... 10
     *The Connection Between the Mind, Body, and Energy System* ........................................................................... 10
   TRAUMA STORED IN THE BODY ....................................................... 12
   FINAL THOUGHTS .......................................................................... 14

**CHAPTER 2: ELEVATING YOUR SELF-CONCEPT** ...................... 15
   UNDERSTANDING SELF-CONCEPT: A PATH TO HEALING ....................... 15
     *Defining Self-Concept* ........................................................ 16
     *The Importance of Self-Concept* ........................................ 17
   EXERCISE: HOW TO ASSESS YOUR SELF-CONCEPT .............................. 18
     *Reflect on Your Beliefs* ....................................................... 18
     *Evaluate Your Self-Esteem* ................................................. 18
     *Compare to Your Ideal Self* ................................................ 19
   LIMITING BELIEFS AND HOW THEY HOLD US BACK .............................. 19
     *How Are Limiting Beliefs Formed?* ..................................... 20
     *What Amplifies Limiting Beliefs?* ....................................... 21
     *How Limiting Beliefs Hold Us Back* ................................... 22
     *Why We Feel "Chained" by Limiting Beliefs* ...................... 26
   EXERCISE: IDENTIFYING AND RELEASING LIMITING BELIEFS .................. 27
     *Step 1: Create a Safe Space* ............................................... 28
     *Step 2: Reflect on Your Beliefs* ........................................... 28
     *Step 3: Identify Limiting Beliefs* ......................................... 30
     *Step 4: Challenge Your Beliefs* .......................................... 31
     *Step 5: Affirm and Visualize* ............................................... 32
     *Step 6: Practice Self-Compassion* ...................................... 33
     *Step 7: Energy Healing Practices* ....................................... 33
     *Step 8: Reflect and Adjust* .................................................. 33
   ASSESSING YOUR OWN MENTAL, EMOTIONAL, AND PHYSICAL HEALTH ....................................................................................... 34

*Assessing Your Mental and Emotional Health* ........................ 34
　　*Assessing Thought Patterns and Emotional Triggers* .............. 35
　　*Taking Stock of Day-to-Day Behaviors* ................................. 38
　EXERCISE: TAKING STOCK OF YOUR PHYSICAL HEALTH........................ 41
　　*Step 1: Create a Calm Environment* ..................................... 41
　　*Step 2: Body Scan* ............................................................. 42
　　*Step 3: Reflect on Emotional Connections* ............................ 43
　　*Step 4: Journaling* ............................................................. 45
　　*Step 5: Set an Intention for Healing* ..................................... 46
　　*Step 6: Daily Practice* ........................................................ 47
　CHOOSING HEALTH, HAPPINESS, AND PROSPERITY ............................ 47
　　*How Do You Think About Yourself?* ..................................... 47
　　*How Do You Nurture Yourself?* ............................................ 48
　　*How Do You Treat Yourself?* ............................................... 48
　　*How Do You Take Care of Yourself Daily?* ............................. 48
　　*The Impact on Health and Happiness* .................................. 49
　　*Self-Concept and Self-Treatment* ........................................ 49
　　*Choosing Happiness and Health* ......................................... 49
　　*Resistance to Health and Happiness* ................................... 50
　　*Creating Aligned Habits, Behaviors, and Belief Systems* ........ 51
　YOU AND YOUR BODY INTUITIVELY KNOW HOW TO HEAL ..................... 51
　　*The Brain-Body Connection* ................................................ 52
　　*The Science of Trauma Storage* .......................................... 52
　　*Healing Through Neuroplasticity* ......................................... 53
　AUTHOR'S STORY ........................................................................ 55
　FINAL THOUGHTS ........................................................................ 61

**CHAPTER 3: EMOTIONAL FREEDOM TECHNIQUE (EFT) TAPPING ................................................................................. 63**

　WHAT IS EFT TAPPING? ............................................................... 63
　　*The History of EFT* ............................................................. 63
　　*How Does EFT Work?* ......................................................... 64
　　*Who Can Benefit From Using EFT?* ...................................... 65
　SCIENTIFIC EVIDENCE SUPPORTING EFT .......................................... 66
　KEY FOCAL POINTS FOR TAPPING .................................................. 68
　WHY DOES TAPPING WORK? ......................................................... 70
　WHAT TO EXPECT ........................................................................ 71
　STEP-BY-STEP GUIDE FOR IMPLEMENTING EFT ................................. 73
　　*Step One: Preparation* ....................................................... 75
　　*Step Two: Self-Acceptance Statements* ............................... 76
　　*Step Three: Identify the Core Issue and Begin Tapping* .......... 76

Step Four: Post-Tapping Reflection ........................................ 77
INTEGRATING EFT TAPPING INTO DAILY LIFE ........................................ 78
LAURA USES EFT TO RESOLVE HER PANIC ATTACKS ............................ 79
CHRISTINE USES EFT TO HELP HER ANXIETY ...................................... 81
FINAL THOUGHTS ................................................................................ 84

## CHAPTER 4: AN IN-DEPTH EXPLORATION OF PSYCH-K ............ 86

WHAT IS PSYCH-K? ............................................................................. 86
  *The Core Principles of PSYCH-K* ........................................... *87*
  *The Seven Methods of PSYCH-K* ........................................... *88*
BENEFITS OF PSYCH-K ....................................................................... 90
  *Julie's Story* ............................................................................. *92*
THE SCIENCE BEHIND PSYCH-K ......................................................... 93
  *The Power of Belief* ................................................................ *95*
  *Neuroscience: The Brain-Body Connection* ......................... *95*
  *Kinesiology and Muscle Testing: The Body's Lie Detector* ....... *96*
  *A Step-by-Step Guide to Muscle Testing* .............................. *98*
IDENTIFY LIMITING BELIEFS: UNCOVER WHAT'S HOLDING YOU BACK ....... 99
  *Recognizing Patterns of Thought: The First Step to Freedom* .. *99*
  *Practical Exercises for Identification: Let's Get to Work* ....... *100*
GUIDED SESSIONS: JOSH'S STORY WITH PSYCH-K .......................... 102
REFLECTION AND JOURNALING EXERCISE: YOUR POST-SESSION MOMENT
................................................................................................... 104
PSYCH-K BALANCE SESSION FORM .................................................. 105
  *Sample Goal Statements for PSYCH-K Balance* ................. *110*
IMPORTANT CONSIDERATIONS FOR PSYCH-K ................................... 110

## CHAPTER 5: THE HEALING WORLD OF REIKI ......................... 114

AN OVERVIEW OF REIKI ................................................................... 114
  *The Ethical Framework* ....................................................... *115*
  *How Reiki Works* ................................................................. *115*
COMMON REIKI MYTHS DEBUNKED ................................................. 116
BENEFITS OF REIKI HEALING ............................................................ 118
  *Releasing Suppressed Emotions* ........................................ *118*
  *Physical Healing* .................................................................. *120*
  *Reiki and Relaxation* ........................................................... *122*
CONSIDERATIONS WHEN PRACTICING REIKI .................................... 124
JAMES' STEP BY STEP REIKI SESSION .............................................. 125
  *Step 1: Pre-Session Preparation* ........................................ *126*
  *Step 2: During the Session* ................................................. *126*
  *Step 3: Post-Session Integration* ........................................ *127*

    Step 4: Enhancing the Experience .................................. 128
    CAN I DO REIKI ON MYSELF? ........................................... 130
    FINAL THOUGHTS .............................................................. 132

**CHAPTER 6: SOMATIC EXPERIENCES ................................ 133**

    WHAT IS SOMATIC HEALING? ........................................... 133
    TYPES OF SOMATIC THERAPIES ...................................... 134
        Somatic Experiencing (SE): Shaking Off the Stress ............. 135
        Sensorimotor Psychotherapy: Your Body Remembers ........ 138
        Accelerated Experiential Dynamic Psychotherapy (AEDP):
        Healing Through Connection .............................................. 142
        Eye Movement Desensitization and Reprocessing (EMDR):
        Rewiring Your Brain ............................................................ 145
        Polyvagal Theory ................................................................ 149
    THE BENEFITS OF SOMATIC PRACTICES ........................... 152
    THE EFFECTIVENESS OF SOMATIC PRACTICES ................. 154
    INTEGRATING SOMATIC PRACTICES INTO DAILY ROUTINES ... 156
        Post-Activity Care .............................................................. 158
    FINAL THOUGHTS .............................................................. 158

**CHAPTER 7: POLARITY THERAPY ...................................... 161**

    AN INTRODUCTION TO POLARITY THERAPY ....................... 161
    THE MAIN GOAL OF POLARITY THERAPY .......................... 162
    HOW DOES A PRACTITIONER BECOME CERTIFIED? ........... 163
    THE FOUR PRINCIPLES OF POLARITY THERAPY ................ 163
        Counseling: The Mind-Energy Connection ........................ 164
        Bodywork: Freeing the Flow ............................................... 164
        Nutrition: Feeding Your Energy .......................................... 165
        Exercise: Moving Your Energy ........................................... 165
    A POLARITY SESSION UP CLOSE ..................................... 166
        The Interview: Discussing Charles' Needs ........................ 166
        Assessing Charles' Energy State ...................................... 167
        Applying Polarity Therapy Techniques .............................. 167
        The First Month: Charles' Journey ..................................... 168
    POLARITY THERAPY AT HOME .......................................... 169
        Keeping Your Body Balanced: The Squat ......................... 170
        Ridding Yourself of Stress: The Woodchopper ................. 171
        Proper Nutrition and Staying Balanced ............................. 171
    IS POLARITY EFFECTIVE? ................................................ 173
    FINAL THOUGHTS .............................................................. 174

## CHAPTER 8: FINDING STILLNESS THROUGH BREATHWORK ........................................................................ 176

BREATHWORK FUNDAMENTALS: BREATHE IN, BREATHE OUT, HEAL ........ 176
THE ROLE OF BREATH IN HEALING ................................................. 178
- Basic Mechanics of Breathing ............................................. 179
- Importance of Intentional Breathing ................................... 180

THE BENEFITS AND SCIENCE BEHIND BREATHWORK ........................... 182
- Physiological Benefits: Relax Your Body, Revive Your Life ..... 182
- Psychological Benefits: Healing From the Inside Out ........... 183

DIFFERENT BREATHWORK TECHNIQUES ........................................... 185
- Diaphragmatic Breathing: Your Foundation for Healing ........ 185
- Boxed Breathing: Finding Your Rhythm ............................... 186
- Alternate Nostril Breathing: Balancing Mind and Body ......... 187
- Clarity Breathwork: Emotional Release in Action ................. 188

GUIDELINES FOR PRACTICING BREATHWORK ..................................... 190
- Creating a Safe Space for Practice ...................................... 190
- Setting Your Intention ........................................................ 191
- Consistency and Patience .................................................. 191
- Journaling and Reflection .................................................. 192

FINAL THOUGHTS ........................................................................ 193

## CHAPTER 9: MINDFULNESS AND MEDITATION ....................... 194

THE ESSENCE OF MINDFULNESS ..................................................... 194
- Definition of Mindfulness .................................................. 195
- Historical Context ............................................................. 195

MINDFULNESS IN HEALING ........................................................... 196
MINDFULNESS TECHNIQUES .......................................................... 198
- Mindful Eating With Patti .................................................. 198
- Body Scan With Patti ........................................................ 199

BENEFITS OF ADOPTING MINDFULNESS ........................................... 200
- Stress Reduction: Mindfulness as a Soothing Pause Button ............................................................................ 200
- Emotional Regulation: Becoming the Calm in Your Own Storm ............................................................................... 201
- Improved Focus and Clarity: Sharpening the Mind's Lens .... 201
- Enhanced Relationships: Showing Up Fully in Every Interaction ....................................................................... 202

DIFFERENT METHODS OF MEDITATION ............................................ 203
PRACTICES TO INTEGRATE MINDFULNESS IN DAILY LIFE ....................... 205
- Mindful Walking ............................................................... 205

    *Mindfulness Reminders: Nudging Yourself to Be Present*..... 206
    *Journaling: Writing Your Way to Mindfulness*...................... 207
  FINAL THOUGHTS ................................................................... 207

## CHAPTER 10: SUPPORTIVE HABITS AND PRACTICES ............ 209
  CREATING A SLEEP ROUTINE................................................... 209
    *Importance of Sleep Hygiene*............................................. 210
    *Techniques for Better Sleep*............................................... 210
    *Addressing Sleep Issues* ..................................................... 211
    *Establishing Calming Pre-Sleep Rituals*............................. 212
  REDUCING STRESS EFFECTIVELY........................................... 212
    *Understanding Stress: The Body-Mind Tango*..................... 213
    *Mind-Body Techniques: Instant Calm Hacks* ...................... 213
    *Creating a Personal Stress-Relief Toolbox: Your Custom Kit* ......................................................................................... 215
    *Setting Boundaries: The Power of "No"* .............................. 216
  INCORPORATING PROPER NUTRITION AND EXERCISE......................... 217
    *Nutrition for Mental Health: Food That Feeds Your Feel Good Energy*....................................................................... 218
    *Creating Balanced Meals: Ditch the Guilt and Love Your Plate* .................................................................................... 219
    *Integrating Movement Into Daily Life* ................................. 219
  FOSTERING HEALTHY RELATIONSHIPS ............................................. 220
  FINAL THOUGHTS ................................................................... 222

## CHAPTER 11: MODALITY CHART ............................................ 223

## CONCLUSION ...................................................................... 225

## BONUS RESOURCES ............................................................ 229

## PLEASE LEAVE US A REVIEW ................................................ 231

## GLOSSARY .......................................................................... 233

## RESOURCES ........................................................................ 237

## REFERENCES ...................................................................... 239

Trigger Warning: This book explores multiple energy healing modalities aimed at helping you heal from trauma. Throughout these pages, we will look at topics related to trauma, emotional pain, and past experiences that may be distressing or triggering for some readers. The content is intended to guide you through healing, but it may also bring up difficult emotions or memories.

Please take care of yourself as you read, and remember that it's okay to pause, seek support, or skip sections if you need to. Your well-being is paramount, and it's important to proceed at your own pace. If at any point you find the material overwhelming, consider reaching out to a mental health professional for additional support.

# About the Author

Emmy Violet is a passionate advocate for holistic healing and self-discovery, a path she welcomed after dealing with her own health journey through the complexities of autoimmune challenges. Faced with a barrage of unexplained symptoms and the limitations of traditional medical interventions, she chose to redefine her health on her own terms, focusing on empowerment and self-love. (Pen Name) embraced personal responsibility and integrated mindful practices, and learned to truly listen to her body and build wellness from within.

Her quest wasn't just about healing; it was about change. Through mindful techniques, energy healing, and a deep commitment to self-awareness, [Pen Name] discovered the power of creating a life filled with strength, empowerment, and purpose. She believes that true healing involves not just the body but the mind and spirit as well.

In her writing, [Pen Name] shares the insights and wisdom she's gathered along the way, aiming to guide others on their own healing path. She encourages you to take charge of your well-being, to trust in your inner wisdom, and to find pure bliss—even humor—in the face of life's challenges. Her mission is to inspire others to begin their adventure of self-discovery, offering them the tools to empower themselves and change their lives with grace, laughter, and love.

# Introduction

Have you ever felt like your emotions are all over the place, and you have no idea why? Or maybe you've noticed patterns that seem to keep you stuck in the same old ruts, regardless of how hard you try to move forward. If so, you're not alone. Nearly 70% of adults in the U.S. have gone through some kind of traumatic event in their lives. Did you know that if trauma is not identified and treated, it can cause long-term health problems like heart disease and autoimmune disorders (Mock & Arai, 2011)?

Many of us carry emotional and mental baggage, trauma that we don't even realize we're lugging around. This book aims to shed light on the hidden burdens stored in our bodies and energy fields, affecting us in ways you might never have imagined.

Trauma isn't just a memory or a passing feeling. Imagine it as a quirky little weight that finds a cozy spot not just in your mind but all over your body, showing up in the form of chronic pain, inflammation, mental stress, anxiety, and even the occasional cloud of sadness. Surprising, right? Well, what if I told you this invisible buddy can have a say in how you feel and act every day?

Trauma doesn't just chill in your thoughts; it also loves to make its home in your muscles, your cells, and even the delightful vibrations of your energy field. Think of your energy field as a magical bubble surrounding you, shaping your vibe with yourself and the world. When trauma shakes things up in this bubble, everything can feel a bit off—you might find it tricky to connect with others or feel like your energy's on a perpetual nap!

Now, here's where it gets fascinating. Our body's energy field, often called the aura, plays an essential role in maintaining our health and well-being. Think of it as your personal Wi-Fi signal;

when it's strong and clear, everything works seamlessly. Conversely, when it's weak or cluttered with "energy gunk," you experience disruptions. The good news is that just as we can boost a Wi-Fi signal, we can also clean and amplify our aura through energy-healing practices.

So, what exactly is energy healing? Imagine it as a tune-up for your soul. Energy healing is considered a holistic practice where energy is channeled into you in order to help balance, heal, and remove blockages from the body (Nesci, 2020). Balance, peace, flow, and vitality within the body can be restored and maintained. Energy healing involves various techniques designed to rebalance your energy field. From Reiki and acupuncture to less-known modalities like polarity therapy, somatic healing, and PSYCH-K, these practices aim to release the deep-seated traumas hindering your emotional and physical health.

Everything in the universe is made up of molecules that vibrate at different frequencies. The molecules in our bodies always vibrate, giving off positive or negative energy, and can be balanced or unbalanced, open or closed. When our organs are not energetically aligned and give off low vibrations, it can lead to physical problems like pain, sickness, and disease (Nesci, 2020).

But let's bring this down to Earth. You don't need to become a spiritual guru or spend hours meditating to benefit from energy healing. Simple exercises and adjustments to your daily routine can yield profound shifts. For example, grounding techniques like walking barefoot on grass or practicing mindfulness during your morning coffee can make a considerable difference in how balanced you feel.

Ready to laugh a little while you heal? This book is your all-in-one toolkit, not just to understand trauma but to laugh in its face and tell it to pack its bags. We'll start by exploring trauma—the big, the small, and the sneaky—and how it likes to set up camp in your body without paying rent. You'll get the insider scoop on how trauma impacts your life and, more importantly, how to evict it for good using powerful energy healing modalities.

Let's be honest—many of us wander through life blissfully unaware of the little (or not so little) traumas weighing us down. This book is here to help you go on a self-discovery quest where you'll pinpoint those pesky traumas and figure out how they've been messing with your mojo. The modalities we'll cover aren't just random techniques; they're like a GPS for your healing path, helping you target the specific traumas holding you back.

But that's not all—we're also going to tackle the sneaky ways your self-image can sabotage your health. If you're walking around thinking, "I'm just a tired, sickly person," well, guess what? Your body might just agree with you! The goal of this book is to help you kick those limiting beliefs to the curb and start identifying as the healthy, strong person you're meant to be. We'll explore self-concept, showing you how to rewire your identity to support your health goals.

Of course, it's one thing to read about all this stuff and another thing entirely to actually do it. That's where the rubber meets the road, my friend. This book isn't here to just give you more information to file away. We're going to talk about the challenges and resistance you'll face in trying to make these practices a daily habit and how to handle them.

Think of this book as your personal cheerleader, coach, and therapist rolled into one. You'll get step-by-step instructions for energy healing practices that are as easy to incorporate into your life as brushing your teeth—just a lot more fun and a lot less minty. The goal? To empower you to take control of your healing, feel supported when the going gets tough, and start seeing real, noticeable improvements in your health and well-being.

By the end of this book, you'll not only have a cleansed and balanced energy field but also a healthier self-image and a new lease on life.

As you move through these pages, you'll discover various modalities to explore and integrate into your life. To make it easier for you to keep track of the pros and cons and how to implement each one, I've included a handy chart after the final chapter. This chart is designed to keep all the valuable information in one convenient place so you can refer back to it whenever you need.

Get ready to laugh, heal, and find a more balanced, empowered you—because you deserve nothing less!

Chapter 1:
# The Mind-Body Connection

Understanding the mind-body connection is like discovering that your smartphone has a hidden feature that can turn it into a magical healing device. Just think about it: your thoughts and feelings can affect your physical health. Ever wondered why you get a stomachache before a big presentation or feel a weight lifted off your shoulders after a heart-to-heart chat with a friend? That's your mind-body connection in action. It's the invisible thread linking your mental state to your physical condition, showing us that our inner world and outer experiences are more intertwined than we might have realized.

It is time to explore how your mental and emotional states communicate with your body through energy signals. Here, you'll find practical techniques—like mindfulness and breathwork—that you can incorporate into your daily routine to foster a better balance between your mind and body. Get ready to unlock the secrets of your own inner symphony!

## Understanding the Body's Energy System

The body's energy system is an intricate network that is truly key to our health. At the heart of this system is the electromagnetic field, often called the body's energy field or aura. This field is composed of various pieces, including electric and magnetic energies that interact with each other and our environment (Chhabra & Prasad, 2019). Our body's electromagnetic field is generated by the electrical activity of our cells, especially those in the heart and brain. The heart's electromagnetic field is the strongest and can be detected from several feet away from the body. It functions as a communication system within the body, sending signals that help regulate physiological processes and maintain homeostasis or equilibrium. One of its crucial roles is in regulating emotions and health (Chhabra & PCrasad, 2019).

Can you picture your body like New York City—busy with highways, intersections, and stoplights? Our energy system is made up of components like chakras, meridians, and energy fields. Meridians are essentially those highways through which life energy—often called Qi or Prana—flows. Each meridian is connected to a specific organ and influences various functions, much like how different roads lead to different parts of a city.

Balancing this energy is kind of like tuning a guitar. All it takes is one string to be off, and the whole melody is wrong. A balanced energy system builds resilience and wellness. It now allows your body to heal itself, so you are sick less often and more capable of bouncing back from trauma. For example, people usually find that after practicing energy-balancing activities like yoga or meditation, their mood improves, and their stress levels drop.

So, how do you ensure your energy is flowing freely like a well-oiled machine? That's where practical applications come in. Simple techniques like visualization and breathwork can improve energy flow. Visualization involves picturing your energy moving through your body like a river, cleansing and revitalizing every cell. Breathwork, on the other hand, uses controlled breathing exercises to unblock stagnant energy and rejuvenate your entire system. Imagine yourself sitting comfortably, eyes closed. You take a deep breath in, imagining bright light filling your chest. As you exhale, you visualize dark clouds leaving your body, taking away stress and tension. Easy, right? These techniques require no fancy equipment, just a bit of time and focus.

Speaking of examples, let's throw in a quick exercise: Try sitting quietly for five minutes each day, focusing on your breath. Take deep breaths through your nose, hold for three seconds, followed by an exhale slowly out of your mouth. Picture your breath as a gentle wave washing over you, clearing any blockages and filling you with positive energy. This simple practice can do wonders for your energy flow.

By now, you're probably thinking, "Okay, this all sounds great, but does it actually work?" The answer is a resounding yes! Numerous studies have shown that practices like meditation, breathwork, and energy visualization can lower stress hormones, improve emotional balance, and even boost the immune system (SenGupta, 2020).

Take acupuncture, for instance. This ancient technique works by stimulating specific points along the meridians, helping to restore energy balance. Many people swear by its effectiveness in treating everything from chronic pain to anxiety. Acupressure follows the same principle but uses fingers instead of needles.

And what about Reiki? A modality of energy healing where practitioners use their hands to channel energy into the patient. The intention is to promote relaxation and healing. Many report feeling a sense of calm, peace, and balance after a session. We will jump into this in more detail in a later chapter.

We've come to realize that the energy field's effect on our aura, physical health, and mental well-being is no small matter. Think of the aura as a multi-layered energy blanket wrapped around us, showcasing our physical, emotional, and spiritual vibes. When our energy field is singing in harmony, our aura bursts with vibrancy and expansiveness, a clear signal that all is well in the world. But when disruptions or blockages occur, that aura may resemble a wilted flower—dull and contracted—hinting at some issues that demand a little TLC.

# The Link Between Mind, Body, and Energy System

One thing's for sure: The energy system plays a fundamental role in our overall health and healing. When you understand and tap into this system, you gain a powerful tool for managing your well-being. Whether you're dealing with emotional scars, physical ailments, or just the daily stresses of life, balancing your energy can offer a path to resilience and recovery.

## *The Connection Between the Mind, Body, and Energy System*

The mind-body connection is a dance of intricate interactions where your thoughts, emotions, and physical sensations come together to create the symphony of your well-being.

Your body's response to your mental state is like a fun dance that affects your overall health! When you're feeling upbeat, your body throws a little party with endorphins, making you feel great. On the flip side, if you're feeling down, your body might show it through tension or fatigue.

These systems really love to interact, creating feedback loops. Positivity leads to a loop of well-being, while negative feelings can turn into physical discomfort, creating a bit of a spiral. Imagine these loops as playful cycles where your emotions influence your health, and your health gives a little nudge back to your emotions. For example, feeling happy and relaxed can give your immune system a boost, while stress and limiting beliefs might take the wind out of its sails, making you more prone to getting sick. When you understand these feedback loops, you can break free from the negative cycles and encourage the positive ones. Recognizing this connection gives you the magic power to make smart choices about your emotional and physical well-being!

Let's pause here for a minute to illustrate this with some real-life stories. Take Patti, who underwent a painful divorce. Her emotional turmoil manifested as chronic back pain and insomnia. Traditional treatments didn't help much until she addressed the root cause: her emotional trauma. Through therapy, yoga, and energy healing, Patti began to understand how her suppressed emotions were affecting her body. As she worked through her grief and anger, her physical symptoms gradually subsided. Patti's path underscores the profound impact of acknowledging and healing emotional wounds to achieve physical well-being. Throughout the coming chapters, we will use real-life stories to walk through each modality, allowing you to see if they will work in your everyday life.

Now, let's talk briefly about mindfulness as a tool. Mindfulness practices, such as meditation and breathing exercises, become essential tools in balancing the connection between your mind, body, and energy.

Practicing mindfulness means being fully present in the moment, which helps you become more aware of your emotional and physical states—like realizing your stomach growls when you skip breakfast! For example, during a stressful situation, practicing mindful breathing can help you stay calm and prevent the stress from negatively impacting your body—because nobody wants to turn into a human pretzel. Studies show that mindfulness can improve emotional regulation, enhance cognitive functions, and promote overall health, making you as steady as a rock (Schuman-Olivier et al., 2020).

To illustrate further, imagine you're feeling anxious about an upcoming event. Your heart races, palms sweat, and thoughts spiral. Now, introduce mindfulness. You can begin by zoning in on your breath, paying attention to each inhale and exhale without judgment. You might notice your heartbeat slowing and your mind calming. This simple act of awareness can shift your energy from anxiety to tranquility, demonstrating the powerful interplay between your mind and body. Chapter nine will explore mindfulness in detail and walk you through real-life situations, allowing you to see it in daily interactions.

## Trauma Stored in the Body

Trauma isn't just a mind game; it also leaves little reminders in your body! When something scary happens, your brain and body jump into action like superheroes in a crisis, but sometimes those feelings hang around longer than you'd like. This is why trauma doesn't just stick to your memories; it can show up in the physical world too!

Let's unpack this idea of "stored trauma." It's kind of like your body has a scrapbook of everything stressful you've been through—where each page is a physical reminder! When something intense occurs, your body floods with stress hormones and kicks into gear. Those feelings can settle into your muscles or cause pesky aches if they don't get a proper farewell hug. So, think of your body as a trusted journal, quietly noting down those dramatic moments affecting you.

You might be wondering how you can tell if you're carrying stored trauma. Well, there are common symptoms to look out for. Chronic pain, headaches, gastrointestinal issues, and even seemingly unrelated ailments like frequent colds can be manifestations of stored trauma. By identifying these symptoms, you empower yourself to seek appropriate healing modalities. It's crucial to understand that if you've been through emotional stress and experience persistent physical discomforts, your body might indeed be holding on to more than you'd expect. Research supports the idea that your body keeps score of trauma. Scientists have discovered that traumatic experiences can lead to impaired cognitive functioning due to increased negative effects during trauma-related situations (Kuhfuß et al., 2021).

Imagine your brain as a giant filing cabinet. Usually, it files away experiences in an orderly fashion, but a traumatic event throws everything into disarray. Studies show that not only does trauma impact mental processes, but it also results in observable physiological changes. For instance, brain scans of individuals with PTSD often reveal alterations in brain areas involved in memory and emotion regulation (Bremner, 2006). These findings underscore the deep-seated nature of trauma, affecting both brain function and body systems.

Perhaps you're now asking, "How do I go about releasing this trauma from my body?" Fortunately, several methods are available, many of which we will tackle in this book!

It's important to emphasize the significance of seeking professional guidance if you have experienced deep trauma. While self-help methods can be immensely beneficial, working with a trained therapist who understands this type of trauma is invaluable. Professionals can guide you through therapies, providing a safe space to explore difficult emotions and bodily sensations.

## Final Thoughts

Understanding the connection between your mind, body, and energy is like discovering a secret cake recipe—it just makes everything better. This chapter has whisked you through how these elements interact, showing that your thoughts and feelings don't just float around aimlessly; they take up residence in your body too. You've learned how emotions can make you feel physically sick or supercharged with endorphins, depending on whether they're positive or negative. Perhaps now, when you get butterflies in your stomach, you'll know it's more than just nerves; it's a full-body conversation happening inside you.

So, what's next? Armed with this knowledge, you can start applying simple techniques like mindfulness and breathwork to keep things running smoothly. Think of these practices as mini tune-ups for your system, helping to balance your energy and ease those emotional aches. By embracing this holistic approach, you're not just putting a Band-Aid on the symptoms but getting to the root of the issue. Remember, understanding and nurturing the mind-body-energy connection can turn you into a resilient powerhouse ready to handle whatever life throws your way.

The goal of the next chapter is to gain a great sense of self and understand who you are by taking an inventory of healthcare needs. It is time to turn the page and move forward in your growth and healing journey.

## Chapter 2:
# Elevating Your Self-Concept

Welcome to elevating your self-concept. Here, we look into the profound impact that a strong and positive self-concept can have on your overall health. Our self-concept is the basis on which we build our beliefs, perceptions, and behaviors. It impacts how we see ourselves and how we interact with the world. When it's strong, we feel confident, empowered, and ready to face life when it gets difficult. When it's weak, we face anxiety, self-doubt, and feelings of unworthiness.

The goal of this chapter is to look at the value of a strong self-concept and provide you with genuine tools to assess your current health and emotional state. Together, we'll take an inventory of your self-concept, identifying areas that need extra attention and healing work. This process will help you gain clarity on how your energy system works, allowing you to work with it, not against it.

Are you ready to elevate your self-concept and change your life?

## Understanding Self-Concept: A Path to Healing

When you question, "Who am I?" the beliefs and qualities you use to respond form your self-concept, which is a blend of all the information and viewpoints shaping your identity. It combines how you see yourself, your traits, and your core values.

## *Defining Self-Concept*

Self-concept is essentially how you see yourself. It includes your beliefs about your nature, identity, and how you perceive your role in life. This view is shaped not only by your personal experiences but also by how others perceive and interact with you. In essence, self-concept is the mental and emotional framework that shapes how you think about yourself.

The three components of self-concept were formed by psychologist Carl Rogers (Perry, 2024):

1. **Self-image:** This reflects how you view yourself. It encompasses your physical appearance, your social roles, and your traits. For instance, you might see yourself as a compassionate friend, a diligent worker, or a creative artist. This category also covers how you "think" others view you.

2. **Self-esteem:** This is about how much value you place on yourself. It's your sense of worth and how you feel about your abilities and limitations. High self-esteem means you appreciate and value yourself, while low self-esteem might make you feel unworthy or incapable.

3. **Ideal self:** This represents the person you strive to be. It's a vision of your best self, encompassing your aspirations, values, and the goals you set for yourself.

The closer your self-image aligns with your ideal self, the more congruent and satisfied you feel.

## *The Importance of Self-Concept*

Having a clear and positive self-concept is crucial for several reasons:

- **Self-understanding:** It helps you understand who you are, guiding your decisions and behaviors.

- **Confidence:** It boosts your confidence and helps you face challenges with a positive outlook.

- **Emotional health:** It contributes to emotional stability, reducing the impact of stress and negative emotions.

- **Personal growth:** It allows you to identify areas for growth and work toward self-improvement.

### *Strong vs. Weak Self-Concept*

A strong self-concept means having a well-defined, positive view of yourself. You recognize your strengths and accept your weaknesses without letting them define you. You have a balanced view, understanding that you are capable and worthy.

On the other hand, a weak self-concept comes with self-doubt, negative self-talk, and an overreliance on others' opinions. You may feel uncertain about your identity and struggle with low self-esteem, often perceiving yourself through a negative lens.

# Exercise: How to Assess Your Self-Concept

### *Reflect on Your Beliefs*

Consider how you describe yourself and the attributes you identify with. If you find it difficult to talk or describe yourself, consider your self-talk. Is this typically positive or negative? Consider the patterns in your life, as they can be an indication of your self-concept.

_____
_____
_____
_____
_____

### *Evaluate Your Self-Esteem*

Ask yourself how confident you are in your abilities. Do you feel worthy? Do you trust yourself and your decisions? How do you measure your self-worth? Is it tied to your performance or accomplishments? What parts of your life do you need to improve?

_____
_____
_____

_____

_____

## *Compare to Your Ideal Self*

Who do you want to be? How close do you feel to that ideal version of yourself?

_____

_____

_____

_____

_____

# Limiting Beliefs and How They Hold Us Back

Have you ever heard that little voice in your head saying, *You aren't capable,* or *You're not valuable?* That's a limiting belief. Limiting beliefs are the negative thoughts and attitudes we hold about ourselves and our capabilities. They act as invisible barriers, keeping us from reaching our full potential. Let's look at what they are and how they start.

Limiting beliefs are essentially assumptions about ourselves and our world that we accept as true. They limit us in various ways, from pursuing our dreams to believing in our worth. These beliefs can be about anything—our intelligence, abilities, relationships, or even our health.

Let's check out some examples:
- "I'm not worthy enough for their love."
- "I always mess things up."
- "I don't deserve to be happy."

These thoughts become so ingrained in our minds that they influence our actions and decisions, often without us even realizing it.

## *How Are Limiting Beliefs Formed?*

Limiting beliefs are typically formed through our experiences, especially those from our childhood. Here's how they often take root (Team Asana, 2021):

- **Early experiences and childhood:** During childhood, we are like sponges, absorbing information and experiences from our surroundings. Our parents, teachers, and peers play significant roles in shaping our beliefs. For example, if you were often told that you were not good at math, you might grow up believing that you're inherently bad at it.

- **Repetition and reinforcement:** When a belief is repeated often enough, it becomes reinforced in our minds. If you continually hear negative comments about yourself, you might start to accept them as truth. Over time, these repeated messages form the foundation of limiting beliefs.

- **Traumatic experiences:** Trauma can greatly impact our belief system. If you experience a traumatic event, it can leave a lasting impression on your mind and body. Let's say you were picked on at school. This could result in a belief that you're not capable of facing confrontation or worth friendships. These beliefs then become ingrained, staying with us after the traumatic event is over.

- **Cultural and societal influences:** Society and culture also play a role in shaping our beliefs. We are constantly bombarded with messages about how we should look, behave, and succeed. These societal standards can create limiting beliefs if we feel we don't measure up.

## *What Amplifies Limiting Beliefs?*

Limiting beliefs don't just appear out of nowhere—certain experiences and influences in our lives often amplify them. Here are some key factors that can intensify these negative thoughts (Rhodes & Grover, 2023):

- **Repetitive negative experiences:** When you encounter the same negative experiences repeatedly, it reinforces the belief that these experiences are your reality. For instance, if you've faced rejection in relationships multiple times, you might start believing you're unlovable.

- **Negative self-talk:** The voice and tone you use when talking to yourself have an impact. Constantly criticizing yourself or doubting your abilities strengthens limiting beliefs. Phrases like "There is no way I can get this done" or "I'm not educated enough" become stuck in your mind.

- **Influences from others:** The opinions and words of those around you—family, friends, colleagues—can amplify your limiting beliefs. If someone important in your life frequently puts you down or undermines your abilities, it's easy to internalize those negative messages.

- **Traumatic events:** Trauma has a powerful impact on our beliefs. Whether it's a single traumatic incident or prolonged exposure to stress and adversity, trauma can create and amplify limiting beliefs about your worth, capabilities, and potential for happiness.

## *How Limiting Beliefs Hold Us Back*

Limiting beliefs can be incredibly restrictive, keeping you from achieving your full potential. Here's how they can impact various aspects of your life (Matthews, 2023):

- **Believing in yourself:** Limiting beliefs chip away at your self-confidence. When you are always doubting your abilities, you are less likely to assume risks or take chances that could take you through growth and success.

- **Engaging in self-love and self-care:** Self-love and self-care require you to believe you are worthy of care and attention. Limiting beliefs make you feel undeserving, leading to neglect of your physical, emotional, and mental well-being.

- **Setting goals:** When you don't believe in your potential, setting meaningful goals seems pointless. You might set small, unchallenging goals to avoid failure or avoid goal-setting altogether.

- **Going after what you want:** Limiting beliefs create a fear of failure and rejection, making you hesitant to pursue your dreams. You might convince yourself that you're incapable or deserving of achieving what you truly want.

- **Enjoying success and happiness**: Even when you achieve success, limiting beliefs can make it difficult to enjoy it. You might feel like an imposter, constantly fearing that your success is undeserved and temporary. This prevents you from fully embracing and celebrating your accomplishments.

Limiting beliefs can also trigger a fight-or-flight response or hold us back in terms of health, which can be deeply ingrained and often stem from past experiences, societal conditioning, or even inherited beliefs.

Let's look at some common types of limiting beliefs around health that can keep us stuck in unhealthy patterns or trigger chronic stress responses like fight-or-flight:

- **Fear-based beliefs:**
    - **"I'm not safe.":** This belief can make you feel like you're always in danger, leading to chronic stress and a constant fight-or-flight state.
    - **"The world is dangerous.":** If you believe the world is unsafe, your body may remain in a heightened state of alertness, unable to relax or trust.
    - **"I'll never be healthy.":** This belief can create a sense of hopelessness and keep you from pursuing positive health changes.

- **Scarcity mindset:**
    - **"There's never enough time for self-care.":** Feeling that time is always lacking can prevent you from taking care of your health, leading to burnout.
    - **"There's not enough resources (money, support, etc.) to get better.":** This belief can prevent you from seeking necessary treatments or making lifestyle changes, keeping you in survival mode.

- **Perfectionism:**
    - **"I have to be perfect to be healthy.":** Perfectionism can lead to chronic stress, as the

pursuit of perfect health is unattainable, causing constant disappointment and anxiety.

- o **"If I can't do it perfectly, it's not worth trying."**: This can prevent you from making small, positive changes, leaving you feeling stuck.

- **Self-worth issues:**

    - o **"I don't deserve to be healthy."**: This belief can lead to self-sabotaging behaviors that keep you in poor health.

    - o **"I'm not good enough to prioritize myself."**: This can make it hard to practice self-care, putting your health on the back burner.

- **All-or-nothing thinking:**

    - o **"If I can't do it all, I might as well do nothing."**: This can lead to a cycle of unhealthy habits, where small setbacks lead to giving up on health goals altogether.

    - o **"It's too late to change."**: Believing that you're too old or too far gone to improve your health can prevent you from making any effort at all.

- **Fear of failure:**

    - o **"I'll fail if I try to get healthy."**: This fear can paralyze you, preventing you from even starting on a health quest.

    - o **"Change is too hard."**: Believing that making changes is too difficult can cause you to stay stuck in unhealthy habits out of fear.

- **Inherited or societal beliefs:**
  - **"My family has always been unhealthy, so I will be too.":** This belief can prevent you from breaking generational health patterns, keeping you in the fight-or-flight response of chronic stress or anxiety about your health.
  - **"Women/men/my people aren't supposed to be healthy.":** Cultural or societal beliefs about gender roles, body image, or ethnic predispositions can limit your ability to seek optimal health.
- **Over-identification with illness:**
  - **"I am my illness.":** When someone over-identifies with their illness or condition, it can become part of their identity, making it harder to envision a healthy future or take actions to improve their well-being.
  - **"This is just who I am.":** Believing that you are inherently unhealthy or predisposed to poor health can limit your ability to make lasting changes.

By identifying and challenging these limiting beliefs, you can start to shift your mindset, reduce chronic stress responses, and open up new possibilities for better health and well-being.

## *Why We Feel "Chained" by Limiting Beliefs*

Limiting beliefs can feel like chains holding you back because they create a mental and emotional barrier that seems impossible to overcome. Here's why these beliefs feel so binding (Matthews, 2023):

- **Deep-rooted in the subconscious:** Limiting beliefs are often deeply embedded in your subconscious, formed from early experiences, and reinforced over time. They become a core part of your identity, making them hard to recognize and change.

- **Fear of the unknown:** Changing your beliefs means stepping into the unknown. The familiarity of your limiting beliefs, even though they're negative, feels safer than the uncertainty of new, positive beliefs.

- **Emotional impact:** Limiting beliefs are tied to strong emotions—fear, shame, guilt. These emotions reinforce the belief and make it difficult to challenge and overcome.

- **Confirmation bias:** Your mind tends to seek out evidence that confirms your existing beliefs. This means you're more likely to notice and remember experiences that reinforce your limiting beliefs, creating a vicious cycle.

# Exercise: Identifying and Releasing Limiting Beliefs

Understanding and releasing your limiting beliefs is a crucial step toward healing and personal growth. This exercise is designed to help you uncover the beliefs that might be holding you back and provide you with tools to start transforming them.

## *Step 1: Create a Safe Space*

- **Find a quiet place:** Choose a quiet and comfortable spot where you can focus without distractions.

- **Set the mood:** Light a candle, play calming music, or diffuse essential oils to create a peaceful environment.

## *Step 2: Reflect on Your Beliefs*

- **Journaling prompt:** Write down the following prompt: "What are the beliefs I hold about myself that limit my potential?"

- **Free write:** Spend 10-15 minutes writing whatever comes to mind. Don't overthink it; let your thoughts flow freely. Be honest with yourself.

_____
_____
_____
_____
_____
_____
_____
_____
_____
_____
_____

_____

_____

### Step 3: Identify Limiting Beliefs

- **Review your writing:** Read through what you've written and highlight any statements reflecting self-doubt, fear, or negativity.

- **List your beliefs:** Create a list of these limiting beliefs. Examples might include: "I'm not good enough," "I don't deserve success," or "I'm always going to fail."

_____
_____
_____
_____
_____

## Step 4: Challenge Your Beliefs

- **Question each belief:** For each belief on your list, ask yourself:

  - Is this belief based on facts or assumptions?

  _____
  _____
  _____

  - Where did this belief come from? (A past experience, something someone said, etc.)

  _____
  _____
  _____

  - How does this belief serve me? How does it hold me back?

  _____
  _____
  _____

- **Write new beliefs:** Replace each limiting belief with a positive, empowering statement. For example, "I'm not good enough" can become "I am capable and deserving of success."

  _____
  _____
  _____
  _____

_____

_____

_____

_____

_____

_____

_____

_____

_____

_____

## *Step 5: Affirm and Visualize*

- **Affirmations**: Write down your new, empowering beliefs as affirmations. Repeat them to yourself daily, preferably in front of a mirror. Example: "I am worthy of love and success." It is completely normal, as you start trying to accept new beliefs, to be met with resistance. You can experience imposter syndrome, almost as if you are wearing high heels when you are used to wearing sneakers. At first, it won't feel comfortable, but the more you wear them (and accept your new beliefs), the easier it will be. When you are prepared for the challenges you might face, you can reduce your anxiety and stay the course.

- **Visualization**: Close your eyes and visualize yourself living your life according to these new beliefs. See yourself succeeding, feeling confident, and achieving your goals.

## *Step 6: Practice Self-Compassion*

- **Self-compassion exercise:** Place your hand on your heart and take a few deep breaths. Say to yourself: "It's okay to have these beliefs. I am on a path of healing and growth. I am kind to myself."

- **Gratitude journal:** Choose a bright, colorful journal that resonates with you. Each day, write down three things you're grateful for. This helps shift your focus from negativity to positivity.

## *Step 7: Energy Healing Practices*

- **Meditation**: Spend a few minutes each day in meditation, focusing on your breath and visualizing a healing light surrounding you, dissolving any negative energy. This will be explored fully in chapter nine.

## *Step 8: Reflect and Adjust*

- **Regular Check-ins**: Set aside time each week to reflect on your progress. Are you noticing any changes in your thoughts and behaviors? Adjust your affirmations and practices as needed.

- **Celebrate wins**: Acknowledge and celebrate your progress. Even during times you feel you aren't making huge progress, even the smallest steps are movement forward.. Every step is a victory.

Remember, identifying and releasing limiting beliefs is an ongoing process. Be patient and compassionate with yourself.

Each step you take brings you closer to healing and living a life aligned with your true potential.

You have the power within you to change your beliefs and create a life filled with joy, confidence, and abundance.

# Assessing Your Own Mental, Emotional, and Physical Health

## *Assessing Your Mental and Emotional Health*

Taking stock of your mental and emotional health is the first step toward healing. It's about understanding where you are right now and what areas need your attention. Here's how you can start:

- **Self-reflection:** Begin by setting aside some quiet time for self-reflection. Find a peaceful spot where you can sit with your thoughts without distractions. This could be in the morning with a cup of tea or in the evening before bed.

- **Journaling:** Writing down your thoughts and feelings can be incredibly revealing. Keep a journal where you document your daily experiences, emotions, and reactions. Note any patterns or recurring themes that emerge.

- **Mindfulness and meditation:** Practice mindfulness to become more aware of your thoughts and feelings in the present moment. Meditation can help you observe your mental state without judgment, allowing you to gain insights into your emotional health.

- **Seek feedback:** Sometimes, those around us can provide valuable insights. Ask trusted friends or family members for their honest observations about your behavior and emotional reactions.

## *Assessing Thought Patterns and Emotional Triggers*

To understand and address your thought patterns and emotional triggers, follow these steps:

- **Analyze thinking patterns:**
    - **Recognize negative patterns:** Pay attention to any negative thinking patterns, such as catastrophizing (expecting the worst), black-and-white thinking (seeing things as all good or all bad), or overgeneralizing (making broad conclusions based on limited evidence).

    - **Replace negative thoughts:** Practice replacing negative thoughts with more positive or realistic ones. For example, change "I always fail" to "Sometimes I succeed, and sometimes I don't, but I always learn."

- **Observe emotional reactions:**
    - **Track your reactions:** Note how you respond to various situations. Do you get easily frustrated,

anxious, or sad? What situations trigger these reactions?

_____
_____
_____
_____

- **Understand the root causes:** Dig deeper to understand why you react the way you do. Often, our emotional reactions are linked to past experiences or unresolved traumas.

_____
_____
_____
_____

- **Monitor recurring emotions and thoughts:**

  - **Daily check-in:** At the end of each day, check in with yourself. What emotions did you experience most frequently? Were there any recurring thoughts?

_____
_____
_____
_____

  - **Pattern recognition:** Look for patterns over time. Are there specific times of day, situations, or people that consistently trigger certain emotions or thoughts?

___

- **Identify emotional triggers:**

  - **List your triggers:** Identify what or who triggers strong emotional responses in you. These triggers could be specific situations, words, or even memories.

  ___

  - **Plan responses:** Once you know your triggers, plan how you can respond differently. For instance, if certain conversations with a coworker trigger anxiety, prepare calming techniques or assertive statements in advance.

  ___

_____
_____

## *Taking Stock of Day-to-Day Behaviors*

Your daily behaviors play a crucial role in maintaining a healthy mind and body. Here's how you can evaluate whether your habits are supportive or detrimental:

- **Create a habit log:** Track your daily activities for a week. Write down everything you do, from the moment you wake up to when you go to bed.

- **Evaluate your habits:** Look at your habit log and ask yourself:

    - **Healthy vs. unhealthy:** Are your habits supporting your mental and emotional well-being? For example, do you start your day with a positive routine, or do you immediately check your phone and feel stressed?

_____
_____
_____
_____
_____
_____

    - **Balance:** Are you balancing work, rest, and play? A healthy lifestyle includes time for productivity, relaxation, and fun.

_____
_____
_____

_____
_____
_____

- **Identify unhealthy patterns:**
    - **Stress-inducing behaviors:** Notice if you engage in behaviors that increase your stress, such as procrastination, overworking, or

- consuming too much caffeine or sugar.

_____
_____
_____
_____
_____

- **Avoidance tactics:** Are you avoiding dealing with your emotions or problems by engaging in distractions like binge-watching TV or excessive social media use?

_____
_____
_____
_____
_____

- **Set goals for change:** Based on your evaluations, set realistic goals to replace unhealthy behaviors with supportive ones. For example, if you notice you're not getting enough sleep, set a goal to establish a calming bedtime routine. It is normal to feel resistant and feel overwhelmed when doing this. Keep in mind that you will learn energy healing modalities to help with this in upcoming chapters.

_____
_____
_____
_____

- **Practice self-compassion:** Remember, this process is about self-discovery and growth, not self-criticism. Be kind to yourself as you make these changes.

When you regularly assess your mental and emotional health by recognizing and addressing limiting beliefs and evaluating your daily habits, you can begin to heal and support your well-being. This requires patience and persistence, but with each step, you'll move closer to a healthier, more balanced life.

# Exercise: Taking Stock of Your Physical Health

Understanding how trauma can be stored in the body is a key step in healing. This exercise will guide you through a mindful reflection on your physical health, helping you recognize any areas of tension, discomfort, or pain that may be linked to past emotional experiences.

## *Step 1: Create a Calm Environment*

Find a peaceful and cozy spot where you can have some quiet time. Get into a comfortable position, sitting or lying down. Start by taking deep breaths to relax yourself. Breathe in deeply through your nose and breathe out slowly through your mouth, allowing your body to unwind with each breath.

## *Step 2: Body Scan*

Close your eyes and bring your attention to your body. Starting from the top of your head, slowly scan down to your toes, taking note of any areas that feel tense, uncomfortable, or painful. Use the prompts below to guide you:

- **Head and neck:** Do you often experience headaches or neck pain? Are there times when your jaw feels tight or clenched?

_____
_____
_____
_____
_____

- **Shoulders and back:** Do you carry tension in your shoulders or upper back? Is your lower back often sore or stiff?

_____
_____
_____
_____
_____

- **Chest and heart area:** Do you feel tightness or discomfort in your chest? Are there times when your heart races or feels heavy?

_____
_____
_____
_____
_____
_____

- **Stomach and gut:** Do you experience frequent stomach aches, indigestion, or other digestive issues?

_____
_____
_____
_____
_____
_____

- **Hips and legs:** Are your hips tight or sore? Do you often feel heaviness or fatigue in your legs?

_____
_____
_____
_____
_____
_____

- **Feet and ankles:** Do your feet or ankles feel sore or swollen by the end of the day?

_____
_____
_____
_____
_____
_____

## *Step 3: Reflect on Emotional Connections*

As you scan each area of your body, consider any emotions or memories that arise. Sometimes, physical discomfort can be linked to specific emotional experiences or traumas. Use the questions below to explore these connections:

- When did you first notice this discomfort or pain?

_____
_____
_____
_____
_____

- Can you recall any specific events or periods of stress that coincide with these physical symptoms?

_____
_____
_____
_____
_____

- How do you feel emotionally when you focus on this area of your body? Are there particular emotions that stand out?

_____
_____
_____
_____

_____
_____

## Step 4: Journaling

Take a moment to write down your observations. Use the following structure to organize your thoughts:

- **Area of discomfort:** Write down the specific area(s) where you noticed tension or pain.

_____
_____
_____
_____

- **Physical sensations:** Describe the sensations you felt (e.g., tightness, aching, burning).

_____
_____
_____
_____

- **Emotional reflections:** Note any emotions or memories that came up during the body scan.

_____
_____
_____

_____
_____

- **Possible connections:** Consider any links between your physical sensations and past emotional experiences or traumas.

_____
_____
_____
_____
_____

## Step 5: Set an Intention for Healing

Based on your reflections, set a healing intention for yourself. This could be something like:

- "I intend to release the tension in my shoulders and let go of the stress that causes it."

- "I aim to understand the connection between my digestive issues and my past experiences, allowing myself to heal."

- "I will be mindful of the emotions that arise when my back pain flares up and address them with compassion."

_____
_____
_____
_____

*Step 6: Daily Practice*

Make this body scan a part of your daily routine. By regularly tuning into your body, you can become more aware of how your physical health is influenced by your emotional well-being. This awareness will prompt healing and releasing stored traumas.

Remember, this exercise is a tool to help you connect with your body and understand its signals. Be patient and gentle with yourself as you explore these connections.

## Choosing Health, Happiness, and Prosperity

Choosing health and happiness is an act of self-love, and it's deeply intertwined with our daily habits, patterns, and belief systems. The way you think about yourself, nurture yourself, and treat yourself shapes your overall well-being. Let's explore this further.

### *How Do You Think About Yourself?*

Your self-concept, or the way you see yourself, plays a significant role in your health and happiness. If you consistently think negatively about yourself, it can lead to a cycle of self-sabotage and unhealthy behaviors. Conversely, cultivating a positive self-concept can inspire you to take better care of yourself. Reflect on your self-talk: Is it kind and encouraging, or is it critical and discouraging? Transforming negative self-talk into positive affirmations can be a powerful step toward choosing happiness.

## *How Do You Nurture Yourself?*

Nurturing yourself means giving yourself the care and attention you need to thrive. This involves both physical care, like eating nutritious foods and getting enough sleep, and emotional care, like allowing yourself to feel and process your emotions. Self-nurturing practices could include mindfulness, meditation, journaling, or engaging in hobbies that bring you joy. By prioritizing self-nurturing, you are sending a message to yourself that you are worthy of love and care.

## *How Do You Treat Yourself?*

The way you treat yourself daily is a reflection of your self-worth. Are you compassionate toward yourself when you make mistakes, or do you punish yourself harshly? Treating yourself with kindness and understanding, especially during challenging times, can impact your mental and emotional health. It's about being your own best friend and supporter.

## *How Do You Take Care of Yourself Daily?*

Daily self-care routines are the building blocks of a healthy and happy life. This includes physical activities like exercise, maintaining a balanced diet, staying hydrated, and getting adequate rest. It also involves mental and emotional self-care, such as setting boundaries, practicing gratitude, and making time for relaxation and fun. Assess your daily habits: Are they conducive to your well-being, or are there areas that need improvement?

## *The Impact on Health and Happiness*

The cumulative effect of your thoughts, self-nurturing practices, self-treatment, and daily self-care habits directly impacts your overall health and happiness. When you align these aspects with your best interests, you create a positive feedback loop that enhances your well-being. Conversely, neglecting these areas can lead to stress, anxiety, and physical health issues.

## *Self-Concept and Self-Treatment*

Your self-concept and the way you treat yourself are foundational to your health and happiness. A positive self-concept empowers you to make healthier choices, while treating yourself with kindness ensures that you maintain those choices. When you value yourself, you're more likely to engage in behaviors that support your well-being.

## *Choosing Happiness and Health*

Choosing happiness and health is about making conscious decisions that align with your values and best interests. It involves recognizing your worth and actively seeking out experiences and behaviors that enhance your life. It means saying yes to what serves you and no to what doesn't.

## *Resistance to Health and Happiness*

Despite knowing what's good for us, we often resist behaviors that support our health and happiness. This resistance can stem from deeply ingrained habits, fear of change, or limiting beliefs about what we deserve. Overcoming this resistance requires self-awareness and a willingness to challenge and change these patterns.

### Creating Aligned Habits, Behaviors, and Belief Systems

To create habits, behaviors, and belief systems aligned with your best interests, start with small, manageable changes. Identify one or two areas you'd like to improve and focus on them. For example, if you want to eat healthier, begin by incorporating more fruits and vegetables into your diet. If you want to reduce stress, start a daily meditation practice.

Additionally, limiting beliefs should be reframed into empowering ones. Instead of thinking, "I don't deserve happiness," try, "I am worthy of happiness and will take steps to achieve it."

Choosing your health and happiness is a path that requires ongoing commitment and self-reflection. It's about creating a life that supports your well-being and allows you to thrive.

Embrace the process with compassion and patience, and celebrate each positive change you make. You deserve a life filled with health and happiness, and it all begins with the choices you make today.

# You and Your Body Intuitively Know How to Heal

When it comes to healing from trauma, whether it's the deep wounds of a life-altering event or the accumulated stress from a string of smaller incidents, our bodies and minds possess incredible abilities. Think of your body as a finely tuned instrument, designed not only to survive but to thrive, even in the face of adversity. The brain and body work together in an extraordinary way, and understanding this partnership is the key to unlocking your healing potential.

## The Brain-Body Connection

Your brain is the command center of your body, orchestrating everything from breathing to your most complex thoughts and emotions. But it's not just sitting up there in your head, detached from the rest of your being. It's in constant communication with every cell in your body through an intricate network of nerves, hormones, and chemicals. This communication network is known as the mind-body connection, and it plays a pivotal role in how we process and heal from trauma (Chu et al., 2022) .

## The Science of Trauma Storage

Trauma can get "stuck" in your body, a concept backed by both ancient wisdom and modern science. When you experience something traumatic, your body reacts with a fight, flight, or freeze response. This response floods your system with stress hormones like cortisol and adrenaline, preparing you to deal with the threat. But if the trauma isn't fully processed, those stress hormones can linger, and the emotional pain can manifest as physical symptoms. This can range from chronic pain and fatigue to digestive issues and even autoimmune disorders.

In Dr. Bessel van der Kolk's book, he explains how traumatic experiences can alter the brain's structure and function, particularly in areas like the amygdala (which processes fear and emotions) and the prefrontal cortex (responsible for reasoning and self-control). This alteration can keep you stuck in a state of hypervigilance or emotional numbness (van der Kolk, B., 1994).

## *Healing Through Neuroplasticity*

Here's where the good news comes in: Your brain is not fixed in its ways. It has a remarkable ability to change and adapt—a phenomenon known as neuroplasticity. This means that even if trauma has altered your brain and body, you have the power to rewire those changes and heal (Chu et al., 2022).

Neuroplasticity allows you to create new neural pathways and strengthen them through practice and positive experiences. This can be as simple as engaging in mindfulness, practicing gratitude, or even physical exercise, which releases endorphins and promotes brain growth. Techniques like the Emotional Freedom Technique (EFT), yoga, meditation, and breathwork can also help you tap into your body's innate healing abilities, calming your nervous system and helping to release stored trauma.

In essence, your brain and body are your greatest allies in the path toward healing. They are equipped with an incredible capacity to recover, adapt, and thrive.

When we make a conscious decision to heal, we set off a chain reaction within our brain and body. It's as if we're sending out an invitation for change, and our brain eagerly RSVPs by beginning to reroute old, unhelpful patterns into more positive and constructive ones.

For instance, if you decide to challenge a long-held belief that you're not worthy of love, you're not just making a mental shift; you're also signaling to your brain that it's time to update its operating system. This conscious shift encourages the formation of new neural connections that align with your new, healthier beliefs. Over time, as you reinforce these beliefs through actions and choices—like practicing self-care, setting boundaries, or seeking supportive relationships—your brain strengthens these pathways, making them more automatic and less effortful. This interplay doesn't just happen in the brain. Our body, especially our nervous system, is deeply influenced by our mental and emotional states. When we commit to healing, we often adopt new behaviors and practices that support this process, such as mindfulness, meditation, or physical activity. These practices help regulate our nervous system, reducing the stress response and allowing us to access a more relaxed, healing state.

For example, when you practice mindfulness, you teach your body to be present in the moment, reducing the impact of stress and anxiety. This helps to calm the nervous system, which can otherwise stay stuck in a fight-or-flight response due to trauma. As your body learns to relax and feel safe, it sends signals back to the brain, reinforcing the belief that you're okay and capable of healing. It's like a feedback loop of positivity—your actions create physical changes, which then support further positive actions.

Humor can play a role here too. Laughing and finding joy in small things can be incredibly healing. It's a way to signal to your brain and body that there's room for lightness, even amid challenges. This isn't about ignoring the tough stuff but rather balancing it with moments of levity that can make healing feel more manageable.

In essence, your personal commitment to healing is like setting the GPS on a road trip. It directs your brain and body toward a destination of well-being, guiding every thought, action, and reaction along the way. When you decide to change behaviors, challenge old patterns, and nurture beliefs that support healing, you're not just passively waiting for time to heal wounds. Instead, you're actively participating in your recovery, empowering your brain and body to work in harmony, creating a more resilient and joyful version of yourself. So, keep steering the course, knowing that every small step is a signal to your system that you're on the path to healing—and that's worth celebrating

## Author's Story

My healing began a few years ago when I started experiencing symptoms that stumped both me and my doctors. I had a cough that lingered for months with no cold in sight, swollen salivary glands, random bouts of fatigue, and mysterious inflammation that seemed to play hopscotch across my body. One day it was my knee, swollen and stiff to the point where walking brought pain, only for the swelling to vanish as suddenly as it had appeared. Another day, I woke up with an eye so swollen it decided to close itself off to the world for a couple of days. These symptoms would come and go like uninvited guests at a party, and after months of this merry-go-round, I finally got some blood work done.

The results? An autoimmune disease. My doctor referred me to a specialist, who handed me a prescription for some heavy-duty steroids. At that moment, I felt like I had hit rock bottom. The thought of being chained to medication for life, with side effects that sounded worse than the disease itself, was terrifying. The idea of a diminished quality of life, compounded by new problems courtesy of the meds, felt like a fate worse than death.

One night, in my desperation, I dusted off a Bible that a nun had gifted me at my high school graduation—a Bible that had been more decorative than functional over the years (seriously, the thing was covered in dust). I opened it randomly, and my eyes landed on a verse about renewing your mind: "Be transformed by the renewing of your minds (*Romans 12:2 In-Context*, n.d.)". And just like that, something shifted inside me. Even though nothing in my external world had changed, I felt a newfound sense of peace. You know that feeling when you read something and think, *Wow, that was written just for me.* That's exactly what happened. It got me thinking—what if our purpose here on this planet is change? And if that's the case, what exactly are we here to transform and transcend? For me, it became clear: I was here to transcend fear and limiting beliefs, and this health issue was life's way of nudging me to grow.

I started exploring my beliefs about health. Was I seeing myself as a healthy person or as someone destined to be dragged down by age and illness? In the months leading up to my diagnosis, I had unknowingly identified as being a helpless victim. But guess what? I learned that I could choose again—I could choose to be the kind of person who takes responsibility for her life and her experiences.

Now, I know that "taking responsibility" can be a triggering phrase for some. It's not about blaming yourself or thinking you somehow "created" your illness. It's about recognizing that you're a powerful creator and that what you focus on and identify with shapes your reality. It's not about effort or hard work; it's about stepping into your power, gaining clarity about what you want, and taking inspired action toward it.

I had spent so long living in fear and dread—dreading the next doctor's visit, dreading the next diagnosis. But after that night with the Bible, I noticed a shift. I stopped living in fear and started feeling a sense of calm and well-being. It was so empowering to detach from the outcome and realize that how I felt didn't have to depend on my external circumstances. I could sit with something unresolved and still feel peaceful.

I also began redefining what health meant to me. I used a technique called PSYCH-K to balance the goal statement, "Every cell in my body is perfectly healthy." It may sound delusional to believe I'm healthy when my symptoms say otherwise, but that's the beauty of transformation. I realized I could choose health for myself—no, scratch that—I could *decide* to be healthy. (Fun fact: the word "decide" literally means to cut out all other options.)

When I accepted health as my new reality, I started seeing any information that contradicted it as either temporary or incorrect, or as something meant to teach me a lesson. Another big shift was learning to sit with what is, even if it wasn't ideal, and remove any judgment from it. This helped me release resistance to what I was experiencing, and suddenly, the present didn't feel so antagonistic.

This healing led to a path of self-discovery. And let me tell you, self-discovery is a self-love adventure. Because when you truly discover who you are, you can't help but fall in love with yourself. (Cue the mic drop moment!) The Romans said, "Know thyself." We can't change what we don't know. Understanding who we are is the first powerful step in healing and living a fabulous life.

I learned some valuable lessons along the way. Sure, I still get the occasional bout of inflammation or fatigue, but now it has a different meaning. I see it as my body's way of signaling that I need to slow down, reduce stress, or practice some self-care. Our bodies, in their infinite wisdom, are always trying to heal. My job is to create an optimal environment for that healing to take place—by nourishing it with healthy foods, staying hydrated, and cutting out toxic junk (both in my diet and in my environment). I also changed the way I viewed doctors. I used to put them on a pedestal, thinking I had to follow their orders without question. But I brought them down from that pedestal and started seeing them as partners.

They have a wealth of knowledge, but ultimately, I'm the one who decides what's best for me. Case in point: When my doctor followed up with me about the steroids, I told her I hadn't taken them and didn't plan to. She was alarmed, of course, but my gut told me I didn't need the medication. And you know what? When you follow your intuition, even without evidence, you might not always feel at ease, but you'll always be right.

I sought a second opinion at the Mayo Clinic, where the diagnosis was the same, but the treatment was entirely different. No prescriptions, just a focus on rest, stress reduction, a healthy diet, and exercise. Fast forward five years, and I'm still not on any medication. I occasionally experience symptoms, but they're fewer and far milder. I've learned that stress and imbalance trigger them, so I've become more mindful of staying out of the chronic fight-or-flight mode that sneaks up on us in our busy lives.

One small habit that made a big difference was setting a reminder on my watch to take a few deep breaths and smile every hour. At first, it seemed silly to interrupt whatever "important" thing I was doing (let's be honest, probably scrolling through social media) to take a few breaths. But I reminded myself that nothing was more important than those breaths. Over time, I noticed that I was habitually taking long, deep breaths, filling my cells with energy and life force, and regulating my nervous system.

It was surprising to me that for the same symptoms, I received two very different prescriptions. Doctors are amazing, dedicated people, but the system isn't designed to emphasize prevention or holistic healing. (Can you imagine going to your doctor and having them walk you through an energy healing session? Now, that would be something!) Instead, the focus is often on managing disease rather than curing it.

I started to trust the process and allowed new things to unfold and incorporate holistic practices into my life. But it wasn't easy—I encountered resistance every step of the way. I visited a dietitian, hoping to improve my eating habits, and walked away feeling discouraged because the advice I got was the same generic stuff you could find with a quick Google search. It took me a full year to actually change my habits and incorporate healthy ingredients into my diet.

Knowing what to do and actually doing it are two very different things, and I learned that the hard way. But here's what worked for me: I identified the tiny habits that would have the biggest impact on my health and well-being, made them visible, removed resistance, and gave myself an instant reward. For example, I wanted to drink more water with electrolytes every day. So, I made it a ritual to fill my favorite glass with water first thing in the morning, add electrolytes, and drop in some sliced strawberries, cucumbers, or lemons that I had prepped over the weekend. Drinking that water felt like a treat—a spa-like experience in a glass.

At the end of each week, I took inventory of how I did. Some days, I dropped the ball, and that was perfectly fine. This exercise was about raising awareness, not self-criticism. I made small tweaks the following week to improve. The only requirement was to not give up—to keep at it, even if I felt like I was failing. Eventually, those tiny habits became second nature.

I always tell my son he's my favorite child, to which he responds, "Mommy, I'm your only child." Treat yourself like you would your favorite child. Pay attention to your self-talk because it directly impacts your mental and overall health. Talk to yourself with respect. As you go through your healing, let go of the need for perfection. Don't beat yourself up if you slip up. If your favorite child fell short despite their best intentions, would you scold them? Of course not.

You'd encourage them with love and compassion. Extend that same love to yourself on this healing path because you are worth it.

We often negotiate our health in our self-talk, telling ourselves, *I hope I get healthy*. We set conditions like, *I'll be healthy after this treatment,* or *When I see that specialist,* or *Once I've taken care of everyone else.* And then, when we get bad news from the doctor, we switch to fear and doubt. This back-and-forth doesn't send a clear message to our subconscious mind, which only accepts our predominant thoughts. So, be unwavering in your choice. What you've chosen for yourself is non-negotiable—it's final.

Another thing I noticed was that I seemed to walk around in a state of amnesia, forgetting how powerful I am and giving my power away to people or circumstances. Anytime we're in a state of fear, doubt, or lack, we're forgetting who we are. The game is to remember that we hold the cards. We can choose to change our state, think better, and do an energy healing practice that soothes and calms our nervous system. We can take a deep breath and focus on something that brings us joy.

I've found that energy healing practices have an instant calming effect on my nervous system, pulling me out of fight-or-flight and making me feel better. Over the long term, these practices have helped me uncover many of my limiting beliefs—beliefs that were lurking just below my conscious awareness. It's like peeling an onion. You might think your limiting belief is one thing, only to discover through energy work that it's something entirely different.

# Final Thoughts

As we wrap up this chapter on elevating your self-concept, take a moment to reflect. Think of your self-concept as the roots of a tree. When those roots are deep, strong, and well-nourished, the tree can weather any storm. It stands tall, its branches reaching for the sky, unafraid to grow and expand. But when those roots are shallow or tangled, the tree struggles to stand firm, easily swayed by the winds of doubt and insecurity.

By taking the time to assess your current health and emotional state, you've begun to untangle those roots, giving them the space they need to grow deeper and stronger. It's not always easy to look inward and confront areas that need healing, but every step you take in this direction is a step toward empowerment and self-discovery.

As you continue to work with your energy system, nurturing it with compassion and understanding, you'll find that your self-concept becomes a solid foundation on which you can build the life you desire—like building a house made of marshmallows: sweet yet stable! You'll start to see yourself in a new light—one that's brighter, more resilient, and fully capable of welcoming the challenges and joys that life has to offer.

So, as you move forward, keep this in mind: Your self-concept is the key to unlocking your full potential. It's the foundation of your well-being, the anchor that keeps you grounded in your truth—kind of like that one friend who always remembers where you parked your car! And that, my friend, is a beautiful place to be, like a sunflower in a field of daisies, soaking up the sun and showing off its fabulous petals!

# Chapter 3:
# Emotional Freedom Technique (EFT) Tapping

EFT tapping, short for Emotional Freedom Techniques, is a powerful way to tackle emotional hurdles. Imagine giving your stress and trauma a gentle nudge out of your system by simply tapping on specific points of your body while talking about it. Sounds like magic, doesn't it? This method brilliantly blends modern psychology with the ancient wisdom of Chinese medicine. It's like giving your emotions a soothing spa day right at home. Whether you're wrestling with daily annoyances or dealing with deeper emotional wounds, EFT tapping offers a hands-on way to find relief.

Are you ready to uncover the magic behind this technique and learn how it works? There's plenty of guidance on how to integrate EFT into your daily routine, making sure that you can maintain emotional balance effortlessly. Hold on tight as we start down this path to emotional freedom, one tap at a time!

## What Is EFT Tapping?

EFT is a fascinating and effective psychological acupressure technique, but where did it all begin?

### *The History of EFT*

Craig recognized the effectiveness of Callahan's approach but found that the intricate algorithms and need for specialized training made TFT less accessible to the general public. Determined to create a simplified and user-friendly method, Craig developed EFT by streamlining the tapping sequences and eliminating the need for acupuncture needles. His innovation made it possible for anyone, regardless of their background or experience, to use EFT as a self-help tool or incorporate it into therapeutic practices. Over time, EFT has evolved into a widely accepted technique for managing stress, anxiety, trauma, and even physical pain. Today, EFT is embraced by therapists, coaches, and individuals seeking a simple yet effective way to enhance emotional well-being (Wilkes & Vartuli, 2023).

## *How Does EFT Work?*

So, how exactly does EFT work? It combines gentle tapping on specific meridian points on your body—such as the side of the hand, top of the head, or under the eyes—with speaking about your issues. These meridian points are the same ones used in acupuncture but without the uncomfortable experience of needles.

When you do this, you help to downregulate your nervous system. In simpler terms, you're telling your brain it's okay to relax, thus reducing the intensity of stress or emotional pain you're experiencing. If you've ever found yourself overwhelmed by emotions or physically tense due to stress, this technique offers a straightforward way to regain control and find some immediate relief.

Developed on the principles of ancient Chinese acupressure and combined with aspects of modern psychology, EFT has been proven highly effective for addressing a range of emotional issues. According to research, consistent tapping on these meridian points sends calming signals to the brain, which can reduce cortisol levels—the pesky stress hormone—in your body (Stapleton et al., 2020). One minute, you might be feeling like a pressure cooker about to explode; the next, you could feel significantly more relaxed.

## Who Can Benefit From Using EFT?

EFT tapping isn't just for those steeped in deep emotional pain or dealing with major trauma. It's versatile and suitable for anyone who wants to improve their emotional well-being. Whether you're grappling with day-to-day stress or tackling deeply rooted traumas, EFT provides a pathway to achieve quick emotional relief and long-term healing. Even if you're skeptical, trying it once might surprise you with its effectiveness.

Practitioners love EFT because it's so adaptable. It works well alongside other therapeutic techniques, strengthening the overall treatment experience. For example, a therapist working with a trauma survivor might introduce EFT into their sessions to help break down emotional blockages that make it difficult to address traumatic memories. The dual approach of talking through experiences while simultaneously tapping can often lead to breakthrough moments faster than traditional talk therapy alone.

One key reason for EFT's growing popularity is its simplicity and accessibility. You don't need years of training to get started with basic EFT. Many online resources and tutorials are available to guide you through the initial steps. Plus, you can do it from the comfort of your own home, which is particularly appealing to people who may not have easy access to a therapist or who prefer managing their emotional health privately. Imagine starting your day with a brief tapping session to set a positive tone or ending your day by releasing built-up stress before bed. Over time, you'll likely notice an improvement in your overall emotional resilience and well-being. You'll find yourself better equipped to handle life's chaos without getting bogged down by stress or anxiety.

Many find that EFT complements other wellness practices they're already engaged in. If yoga, meditation, or mindfulness activities are part of your routine, adding EFT can further strengthen your emotional balance. Think of it as another tool in your self-care toolkit. When you integrate tapping into your existing practices, you create a more comprehensive approach to maintaining mental and emotional health.

Another great thing about EFT is that it's not just a feel-good party for your emotions; it throws a little love into your physical health too! Lowering stress and cortisol levels is like giving your body a high-five—it directly boosts your health. Stress can take a wrecking ball to your immune system, leaving you wide open for all sorts of illnesses. So, by dialing down the stress, EFT is like your body's personal trainer, beefing up your immune response and helping you bounce back faster when the sniffles strike.

Just like any good habit, the secret to rocking EFT is sticking with it. You might feel like a new person after just one session, but making it a regular thing really deepens those benefits. Think of it like brushing your teeth—skipping out for weeks won't leave you with a dazzling smile! Consistent EFT tapping is your go-to for keeping emotional stress at bay and your mood high.

## Scientific Evidence Supporting EFT

Scientific research offers compelling evidence for the effectiveness of EFT tapping in trauma recovery and emotional regulation. You're probably wondering, does this really work? Well, let's dive into what the studies say.

First, multiple studies indicate that EFT sessions can lead to reductions in cortisol levels and associated anxiety symptoms. Cortisol is often referred to as the "stress hormone," and high levels can wreak havoc on your emotional and physical health. Research has shown that after participating in EFT sessions, people experience lower cortisol levels, translating into reduced stress and anxiety (Bach et al., 2019). It's like giving your body's alarm system a chance to calm down.

Now, let's talk about the brain. Tapping on specific energy points has been found to influence the amygdala, the part of your brain responsible for processing emotions like fear and pleasure. Targeting the amygdala can help reduce the emotional charge attached to traumatic memories (König et al., 2019). Imagine having a volume knob for your fears and anxieties, and EFT helps you turn it down. In this way, the technique allows you to recall a distressing event without reliving the overwhelming emotions associated with it. This neural rewiring makes it possible for you to handle life without being hijacked by past traumas.

The efficacy of EFT is further validated through comprehensive reviews, which have highlighted significant reductions in PTSD, anxiety, and depression among those who use EFT compared to control groups not using the technique (Feinstein, 2023). Picture two groups: one tapping their way to relief and the other just chilling—and guess which group showed more improvement? Yup, the tappers. Such findings are especially promising for trauma survivors or anyone grappling with emotional and mental health issues.

Research also documents remarkable improvements in PTSD symptoms and overall emotional resilience after several EFT sessions. For instance, veterans suffering from PTSD have seen substantial relief after engaging in EFT. Imagine carrying the weight of your traumatic experiences every day and then, slowly but surely, feeling that weight lift. Participants not only report alleviated PTSD symptoms but also note an increase in their ability to bounce back from future emotional setbacks (Bach et al., 2019). It's like building emotional muscle; the more you tap, the stronger you get at handling what life throws at you.

So, it turns out that those who do EFT tend to feel a lot more relaxed and emotionally stable. You might be thinking, how can just some tapping do all that? Well, picture EFT as a workout for your feelings, kind of like yoga or meditation is for your body and mind. It's like a one-two punch—thinking differently about your issues while giving yourself a little tap dance on your body!

In case you're looking at EFT skeptically, thinking it sounds almost too good to be true, remember that the American Psychological Association and other reputable organizations have recognized its merits. Courses on EFT have been offered for continuing education credits by prestigious institutions like the APA, AMA, and ANCC since the early 2010s (*Expert Training*, 2024). Essentially, the growing acceptance of EFT within mainstream psychology and medicine underscores its credibility.

## Key Focal Points for Tapping

The basic EFT tapping points are scattered all over your upper body, starting from the top of your head down to your wrists. Each point corresponds to a major energy channel or meridian that flows through your body. These points are not picked randomly; they're tied to the ancient Chinese medicine practice of acupuncture but without the needles. Let's look at these more in detail (Anthony, 2023):

- **Top of the head:** At the very top of this tapping process is—you guessed it—the top of your head. This point is known for being a sort of "reset button" for your brain. Tapping here can help calm your mind and bring clarity.

- **Eyebrow:** Moving down to your eyebrow point, this is located right where your brow starts near the bridge of your nose. It's a spot that can help reduce feelings of frustration and overwhelm.

- **Eye point:** Next, you should tap on the side of the eye point, which is right on the bone at the corner of your eye. This spot is excellent for letting go of fears and anxiety.

- **Under eye bone:** Underneath the eye, you'll find another key point. Tap gently here on the bone just under your eye. Got some sadness or regret bottled up inside? This point can help release those emotions.

- **Between top lip and nose:** Sliding down to the area between your top lip and nose, you've got the under-the-nose point. This little space packs a punch in releasing shame and powerlessness.

- **Chin:** Right below that, on the chin, is another powerful spot. Tap here to tackle feelings of doubt and insecurity.

- **Collarbone:** Next up, we have the collarbone point. Just below your collarbone, this point is perfect for alleviating any feelings of worry and stress that seem to weigh heavily on your chest.

- **Underarm point:** Continuing downward, you'll find the underarm point. This is located about four inches below your armpit. It's great for releasing feelings of guilt and entrapment.

- **Wrist points:** Finally, don't forget your wrist points! Gently tap on the inner sides of both wrists together. This helps balance your entire energy system, giving a final sweep to erase lingering negativity.

## Why Does Tapping Work?

Now, beyond knowing where to tap, it's really important to understand why tapping works. When you tap on these meridian points while focusing on negative emotions or memories, what you're doing is sending signals to the amygdala, the brain's panic button. These signals tell your brain it's safe to relax, releasing the grip of stress or trauma (*EFT Tapping Points: 12 Primary Meridian Points Tapping*, 2023).

Imagine carrying around a backpack full of rocks representing every negative emotion or traumatic memory you've ever had. It's heavy, right? EFT tapping is like systematically removing those rocks and lightening your load, one tap at a time. The process allows you to address various issues, whether they stem from childhood trauma, recent stressful events, or generalized anxiety. By tapping on these points, you create an opportunity for emotional freedom, a chance to breathe easier and live lighter.

What's also interesting is how different points can work better for different people. Your best friend might swear by the under-eye point for banishing her worries, while you may find that the collarbone point is your secret weapon against stress. This individuality makes EFT tapping a deeply personalized experience, allowing for unique healing tailored to each person's emotional landscape.

Experimentation with these points might reveal specific preferences. You may find yourself drawn to tap more frequently on certain points than others, and that's perfectly okay. The beauty of EFT is its flexibility and adaptability to individual needs. Some people even develop sequences or routines that specifically address certain emotional states, creating a custom-tailored approach to their healing.

While the technique itself is straightforward, the impact can be profound. The rhythm and repetition of tapping act almost like a mantra, grounding you in the present moment. As you focus on the act of tapping and the sensations it brings, your mind becomes less cluttered with intrusive thoughts and negative emotions. This practice enhances not only relaxation but also promotes a holistic sense of well-being.

## What to Expect

User experiences often add fascinating layers to this understanding. Many people report feeling immediate relief or shifts in their emotional state post-tapping. Some might feel a sense of lightness, relaxation, or even physical sensations like tingling warmth. These responses can vary widely but almost always point toward an overall release of tension and built-up stress.

During and after EFT tapping sessions, you can expect the following:

**During the session:**

- **Focused tapping on specific points:** As discussed, expect to tap on specific acupressure points on the body, typically while focusing on an issue or emotion that needs to be addressed. The practitioner or self-guided instructions will guide you through these points.

- **Verbalizing emotions or issues:** You'll verbally acknowledge the emotions, memories, or issues you want to release. This might include repeating specific phrases that help you stay focused on the problem while tapping.

- **Emotional intensity:** You may experience a temporary increase in emotional intensity as you focus on unresolved feelings. This is a normal part of the process as you work through the issue.

- **Physical sensations:** You might feel tingling, warmth, or other physical sensations as the energy shifts. This can be part of the body's response to the tapping process.

- **Calmness or relaxation:** As the session progresses, you may begin to feel a sense of calm or relaxation, even if you started with intense emotions.

**After the session:**

- **Emotional relief:** Post-session, you might feel a big reduction in the intensity of the negative emotions you were addressing. It is possible to feel lighter and more at peace.

- **Increased clarity:** You may experience mental clarity and a new perspective on the issue you worked on, allowing you to approach it with more balance and insight.

- **Physical relaxation:** The body often responds positively to EFT, leading to a sense of physical relaxation and tension relief.

- **Ongoing processing:** In the hours or days after a session, you may continue to process the emotions or memories that came up during tapping. This could lead to further emotional release or insight.

- **Improved emotional resilience:** With repeated sessions, you might find that you become more resilient to stress and better able to manage your emotions when life brings chaos.

- **Varying results:** The impact of EFT varies for each person and from session to session. You may experience immediate shifts or may need several sessions to notice any changes.

These expectations can help you approach EFT with an open mind, allowing the process to work through both immediate and long-term benefits.

## Step-By-Step Guide for Implementing EFT

Imagine you're standing in a serene forest, ready to start on an inner quest of healing and emotional freedom—hopefully without tripping over any tree roots! That's the essence of EFT tapping—a path to release trauma and foster well-being, minus the awkward conversations with squirrels.

Let's dive into how you can conduct your own EFT tapping sessions effectively, starting with preparation (don't forget to stretch those fingers!), moving through the tapping procedure, reflecting on your experience (discussing it with your pet goldfish counts!), and finally integrating this practice into your daily life.

Before you start tapping away your worries, it's key to prepare. Think of this as laying the groundwork for a successful session. Begin by setting your intentions.

Take a moment to tune into your feelings. Close your eyes, take a few deep breaths, and let yourself really feel the emotion or issue that's bothering you. This act of "tuning in" guarantees that you're genuinely connected to what you wish to address.

These are pivotal because they acknowledge your current feelings while fostering a sense of self-acceptance. Let's look at some examples:

## *Step One: Preparation*

Before you start tapping away your worries, it's key to prepare. Think of this as laying the groundwork for a successful session. Begin by setting your intentions.

- What do you want to achieve with this session?
- Are you looking to alleviate stress?
- Do you want to reduce anxiety?
- Perhaps you are looking to tackle a specific fear?

Take a moment to tune into your feelings. Close your eyes, take a few deep breaths, and let yourself really feel the emotion or issue that's bothering you. This act of "tuning in" guarantees that you're genuinely connected to what you wish to address.

## Step Two: Self-Acceptance Statements

These are pivotal because they acknowledge your current feelings while fostering a sense of self-acceptance. Let's look at some examples:

- "Even though I feel this anxiety, I deeply and completely accept myself—like accepting a cat in a tutu."

- "I recognize that I am struggling, and I give myself permission to feel this way—after all, even superheroes have bad days."

- "Even when I am overwhelmed, I welcome my imperfections like a fruitcake at Christmas."

- "I accept that it's okay not to be okay sometimes—just like it's okay to eat dessert for breakfast. There's a time and place for everything!"

- "As I handle this challenge, I honor my feelings and trust in my process, even if my GPS keeps trying to re-route me."

- "I fully accept my path and understand that growth takes time—like waiting for that perfect avocado to ripen."

This dual approach helps you acknowledge your emotions without judgment, making it easier to shift them during the tapping process.

## Step Three: Identify the Core Issue and Begin Tapping

Start by identifying the core issue you want to address. Rate its intensity on a scale from 0 to 10, where 10 is the most intense. This will help you gauge your progress throughout the session.

Begin the tapping sequence. As discussed, the basic points include the top of the head, eyebrow, side of the eye, under the eye, under the nose, chin, collarbone, under the arm, and the wrist. Tap gently on these points using your fingertips while repeating your self-acceptance statement. For instance, as you tap on the eyebrow point, you could say, "Even though I feel this anxiety, I choose to release it now."

Give this sequence a go several times—no need to sprint; this isn't a race, after all! Take your sweet time with each point, and let yourself get cozy with the process. Just a heads-up: As you keep going, you might feel your mood do a little cha-cha. Keep tapping until those emotional fireworks fizzle out. And hey, if some surprise issues pop up, just continue to handle them with the same technique until the calm returns.

## *Step Four: Post-Tapping Reflection*

Once you've completed the tapping sequences, it's important to reflect on your experience. Take a moment to reassess the intensity of your original issue—yes, it's time for your emotional performance review! Rate it again on the same scale from 0 to 10. Ideally, you should see a decrease in the intensity. Reflect on any insights or revelations that have emerged during the session. Documenting your experience can be incredibly valuable. Grab a journal and jot down your thoughts, feelings, and any changes you've noticed—think of it as your emotional diary, complete with a "no judgment" policy. This not only helps in tracking your progress but also provides a reference for future sessions. Over time, you'll likely see patterns emerging, helping you understand your emotional triggers better and reinforcing the effectiveness of your EFT practice—like a detective solving the case of the disappearing stress!

## Integrating EFT Tapping Into Daily Life

The beauty of EFT tapping is that it's not just a one-time fix; it can become a part of your daily routine, providing ongoing support for your emotional well-being. To get the most out of EFT, consider incorporating regular tapping sessions into your daily life. You don't need to wait until you're overwhelmed with stress or anxiety. Think of it as a preventative measure. Regular tapping can help you maintain a balanced emotional state and keep stress levels in check.

You can also use EFT before potentially stressful situations. Have a big presentation coming up at work? A challenging conversation you've been dreading? Spend a few minutes tapping to calm your nerves and ground yourself. This proactive approach can make a significant difference in how you handle stressful events. Here are five examples of how to integrate EFT tapping into your daily life with ease. With these quick tapping hacks, EFT can become your go-to tool for handling life's chaos.

1. **Morning stress detox:** Kickstart your day by tapping away any pre-coffee jitters. Spend a few minutes tapping on those magic points, acknowledging your inner Monday-morning-monster, and finish with affirmations like, "I've got this—coffee or not."

2. **Pre-meeting power-up:** Got a big work day ahead? Before you dive in, give yourself a quick tapping tune-

up. Tap away those "what if I trip on my words" fears and replace them with, "I'm as smooth as butter."

3. **Afternoon reboot:** When the dreaded 3:00 p.m. slump hits, skip the extra espresso and go for a tapping pick-me-up. Tap through the afternoon fog, and remind yourself, "I'm powering through this like a boss—no nap required."

4. **Evening emotional unload:** After surviving another day, make tapping part of your wind-down routine. Let go of all the nonsense that's been thrown at you and tap your way to a Zen-like calm with thoughts like, "Goodbye, stress. Hello, Netflix."

5. **In-the-moment chill pill:** When your life gets messy (like a busted pipe or that never-ending family drama), sneak in some taps. Silently acknowledge the chaos and tap your way back to sanity with a mantra like, "I've got this, and no, I won't eat my emotions."

EFT tapping offers you a way to take charge of your emotional health, putting the power of healing literally into your hands—or should I say fingertips! By following these guidelines—preparation, the tapping procedure, post-tapping reflection, and daily integration—you're well on your way to achieving emotional freedom and well-being.

## Laura Uses EFT to Resolve Her Panic Attacks

Imagine struggling with panic attacks and anxiety. Every day feels like a battlefield. This was Laura's reality until she stumbled upon EFT tapping. Laura's path with EFT began out of sheer desperation. Panic attacks had turned her life upside down, making even the simplest tasks feel insurmountable.

Laura had always been a perfectionist, juggling a demanding job, trying to maintain her social life, and taking care of her family. The pressure to perform at her best—always—led to chronic stress that slowly built up over time. The tipping point came when she started waking up in the middle of the night with her heart racing, feeling like she couldn't breathe. What had once been manageable stress spiraled into full-blown anxiety, manifesting as panic attacks that struck without warning.

The everyday things that most people take for granted became monumental challenges for Laura. Grocery shopping? Impossible without feeling lightheaded and overwhelmed by the crowds. Driving to work? A nightmare of sweaty palms and racing thoughts as she sat in traffic, fearing she'd lose control. Even something as simple as replying to emails felt like an insurmountable task—her mind would race with "what ifs," and she'd freeze, unable to take action. These once-routine activities had become her biggest sources of dread, feeding into a vicious cycle of anxiety.

She first heard about EFT from a friend who swore it changed her life. Skeptical but hopeful, Laura decided to give it a shot. Little did she know this decision would become a turning point in her life.

Laura's first EFT session focused on her fear of driving alone, which was a significant trigger for her panic attacks. During the session, a practitioner guided her through tapping specific points while she verbalized her fears. It felt odd at first—tapping on her face and body while repeating phrases about her anxiety. However, after a few rounds, she noticed something incredible.

Her heart rate slowed, her hands stopped shaking, and she felt an unfamiliar sense of peace. It was as if the panic had been siphoned out of her body.

Over the following months, Laura integrated EFT into her daily routine. Each morning before facing the world, she spent ten minutes tapping away her anxieties. Gradually, she found that the panic attacks decreased in frequency and intensity. Tasks like grocery shopping or attending social gatherings no longer seemed so overwhelming. Her experience with EFT gave her a newfound confidence and control over her emotions, helping her reclaim her life.

## Christine Uses EFT to Help Her Anxiety

Christine faced debilitating anxiety following a traumatic car accident. That fateful day left her physically able to heal, but emotionally, she was left scarred in ways she never imagined. The impact of the accident went beyond the visible injuries; it shattered her sense of safety and left her battling a constant state of hypervigilance. Every time she closed her eyes, she was back in that moment—the screeching tires, the deafening crash, the overwhelming fear. Flashbacks would strike at the most unexpected times, making her heart race as if she were reliving the accident over and over again.

Her fear of cars became all-consuming. Just hearing the sound of a car horn would send her into a panic, her breath catching in her throat, her body freezing as if she were bracing for another impact. Christine couldn't even pass by a busy street without feeling the familiar surge of anxiety tightening her chest. The thought of getting back into a car was unimaginable; driving herself was out of the question, and even riding as a passenger felt like an impossible task.

But it didn't stop there. Christine's anxiety extended to her family as well. She became obsessed with their safety, particularly when they were driving. If her husband or children were out in the car, she couldn't rest until she knew they had arrived safely. She would insist that they call or text her the moment they reached their destination. Yep, she became "that" chronic texter who blew up their phones until she received a reply. If they didn't respond quickly enough, her mind would spiral into catastrophic thinking—visions of accidents and worst-case scenarios playing on a loop in her head. She would sit by the phone, her heart pounding, unable to focus on anything else until she knew they were safe.

Nightmares plagued her sleep, filled with images of crashes and chaos. She'd wake up in a cold sweat, her heart racing uncontrollably, struggling to separate the dream from reality. The panic didn't end when she woke up; it lingered, wrapping itself around her day, making it difficult to concentrate on anything other than her fear.

Christine's need for control began to dominate her life. She couldn't help but micromanage every detail of her loved ones' movements (admittedly driving them a bit nuts), especially when it involved driving. She needed to know every step of their journey as if somehow her vigilance could protect them from harm. This overwhelming need to control was her way of coping with the trauma, but it also trapped her in a cycle of anxiety that she couldn't break free from.

Her life had become a series of anxious waiting games, where every honking horn, every missed call, and every traffic report on the radio sent her spiraling into panic and added about six more gray hairs. It wasn't just about the fear of another accident—it was about the loss of control and the constant anticipation of disaster.

After a few months in psychotherapy, it would be her therapist who would recommend EFT. Christine initially dismissed EFT, thinking it was too simplistic for her complex trauma. But her therapist convinced giving it a try, and she agreed.

Christine's EFT path started slowly. At first, she was reluctant to confront the memories of the accident. Tapping on the meridian points felt strange, almost silly. But during one session, as she tapped on her collarbone while talking about the crash, she broke down and sobbed. It wasn't just a release of tears but a release of pain. With each subsequent session, she peeled back layers of trauma. She described feeling lighter, as if the emotional burden was being lifted tap by tap.

As Christine continued with EFT, she noticed profound changes. Over the next six months, the flashbacks became less vivid, and the thought of driving didn't induce panic anymore. She even took short drives with her husband, building up her confidence behind the wheel again. EFT transformed her relationship with her trauma, turning it from an all-consuming monster into a manageable memory.

Personal stories like those of Laura and Christine highlight EFT's accessibility and effectiveness. These narratives don't just showcase success; they provide a roadmap for readers seeking a way out of their emotional turmoil. Through relatable experiences, you can visualize how EFT might fit into your own healing process.

When dealing with intense emotions and traumatic memories, it's easy to feel isolated and overwhelmed. EFT offers a tangible method to address these feelings, helping to foster emotional freedom and resilience. Its simplicity is its strength—the act of tapping combined with verbalizing can create profound internal shifts.

For anyone skeptically standing on the threshold of trying EFT, these personal accounts serve as a gentle push. They underscore that you aren't alone in your struggles and that there are tools like EFT available to help you navigate through them. Whether it's dealing with day-to-day anxiety, overcoming a traumatic event, or managing deep-seated PTSD, EFT has shown time and again that it can offer relief and a path to emotional well-being.

## Final Thoughts

You've made it this far, bravely moving through the ins and outs of EFT tapping. By now, you should have a pretty good handle on how tapping can help release all that pesky emotional baggage. Whether it's tackling daily stresses or diving deep into trauma recovery, EFT offers a simple and effective tool right at your fingertips. It's like having a magic wand for emotional well-being—minus the glitter and obligatory wizard hat.

So, as you step away from this chapter, remember: Your hands aren't just for holding snacks or swiping through social media. They're powerful tools for healing. The beauty of EFT tapping is its accessibility—you don't need any special skills or equipment. Just a bit of time, focus, and those handy tapping points you've learned about. Keep practicing, stay consistent, and soon you'll find yourself tapping away stress and unlocking doors to a happier, healthier you.

Up next will be an introduction to the PYSCH-K method and how it changes your limiting beliefs and your life!

# Chapter 4:
# An In-Depth Exploration of PSYCH-K

This chapter aims to dive into the world of PSYCH-K. We'll start by getting our heads around the basics and figuring out what makes it stand out from other energy psychology techniques. You'll discover the perks of using PSYCH-K, with enough scientific evidence and jaw-dropping case studies to impress even the most skeptical. We'll also chat about some hands-on tools, like muscle testing and the balancing acts we'll do. By the end of this chapter, you'll be ready to try some exercises yourself or team up with a facilitator to unleash the mind-blowing powers of PSYCH-K!

## What Is PSYCH-K?

PSYCH-K, pronounced "sigh-kay," is a relatively unknown but powerful healing modality. It stands out in the field of energy psychology because of its unique approach to transforming limiting beliefs and aligning one's subconscious mind with conscious goals. The name itself combines "psychology" and the letter "K," symbolizing the key to sustainable change.

PSYCH-K is basically your mental gardening tool, helping you pull out pesky weeds of negativity and plant seeds of personal pizzazz for some serious emotional glow-up!

The origin of PSYCH-K dates back to 1988, when it was developed by Robert M. Williams, a psychotherapist deeply invested in understanding how beliefs affect different aspects of our lives. Frustrated by the limitations of traditional talk therapy, Williams wanted a more effective way to facilitate belief change. He combined elements from various fields like neuroscience, biology, and mind-body/spirit integration, resulting in PSYCH-K—a method that looks to bridge the gap between the conscious and subconscious mind (Kylie, n.d.).

## *The Core Principles of PSYCH-K*

Alright, let's dive into PSYCH-K and how it can unlock your body's energy, release trauma, and help you embrace self-worth—without making you feel like you're trapped in a never-ending wellness seminar. Ready to flip the script on those self-limiting beliefs? Great! Let's go.

PSYCH-K isn't your average self-help tool. It's like a makeover for your subconscious, but instead of new shoes, you're getting a fresh mindset. Here's the lowdown:

- **Switch it up:** At the heart of PSYCH-K is a simple yet powerful balance process that helps you switch out those pesky subconscious beliefs like you're swapping out an old, uncomfortable chair for a cozy new one. This is where real change happens—deep in the subconscious, where your mind's autopilot lives.

- **Own your journey:** PSYCH-K also nudges you toward some good old self-awareness and personal responsibility. Yep, you're in the driver's seat of your healing. No more blaming the universe or your cat for everything (though we know they're secretly plotting).

Now that you know the basics, let's get into the juicy stuff—the seven methods of PSYCH-K that make this all possible.

## *The Seven Methods of PSYCH-K*

PSYCH-K uses seven different techniques designed to create positive changes in multiple areas of your life. Let's take a closer look at those now (*What Is PSYCH-K and How Does It Work?*, n.d.):

1. **Self-muscle testing:** Ever wish your body could just tell you what's going on in your mind? Well, PSYCH-K says, "Wish granted!" Self-muscle testing is like having a direct chat with your subconscious, using your body as the interpreter. It's like your body is texting you back, saying, "Hey, here's the scoop!" All you need is a little pressure on these points, some focus, and voilà—subconscious communication, no Wi-Fi required.

2. **Whole brain integration processes:** This one is about getting your brain to play nice with itself. You know how sometimes your left brain and right brain feel like they're arguing at a family reunion? Whole brain integration makes sure both hemispheres are on the same page, ready to create peace and squash that old trauma. Think of it as yoga for your brain—minus the pretzel-like stretching.

3. **Permission protocols:** Unlike some therapies that just barge in and start rearranging furniture, PSYCH-K is all about asking for permission first. This is where you check in with your subconscious and your highest self to make sure everyone's cool with the changes. It's like asking your inner wisdom, "Hey, is it safe to move this couch of beliefs?" If the answer is yes, then you proceed. If not, you adjust accordingly.

4. **Stress transformation:** Ever feel like your body is stuck in a time warp, reacting to present stress as if it's reliving past trauma? PSYCH-K can help hit the reset

button on that. When you learn to change your body's stress response, you can finally take that deep breath and say goodbye to the old triggers that have been running the show. The best part? You get to reclaim your calm and start living like the past is truly behind you.

5. **Belief statements:** Ah, the power of words! In PSYCH-K, belief statements are like little love notes you send to your subconscious. They're simple, positive, and all about you. Think of them as daily affirmations on steroids. These statements reprogram your subconscious to believe in a new reality—one where you actually enjoy learning new things, for example. The trick? Keep them in the present tense because your mind is all about the now.

6. **Action steps:** Now, belief statements are great, but PSYCH-K isn't just about thinking good thoughts while sipping herbal tea. It's about taking action. Action steps are your way of putting those new beliefs into motion. It's like setting up a to-do list for your future self—a future that aligns with your new mindset. Plus, crossing things off that list is just as satisfying as ever.

7. **Specific advanced balances:** For the overachievers out there, advanced PSYCH-K balances take things up a notch. These aren't your regular, run-of-the-mill balances; these are the big guns. Whether it's healing relationships (yes, even with that one ex) or working on deep-rooted beliefs about health and wellness, advanced balances help you tackle the big stuff. There's even a life-bonding balance that deals with the anxiety

around death. If you're ready to go all-in on your healing, this is where it gets real.

## Benefits of PSYCH-K

Imagine this: you're carrying around limiting beliefs—those sneaky little thoughts convincing you you're not enough or you can't achieve what you want. PSYCH-K steps in like your personal belief buster, combining techniques from psychology, kinesiology (that's muscle testing, for those who are wondering), and a bit of neuro-linguistic programming (NLP) magic to help you rewire those outdated beliefs.

Think of PSYCH-K as a remix. It takes the best of various healing and therapeutic disciplines, stirs them up, and creates a technique all about unlocking your potential. Over the years, it's grown from a cool idea into a fully-fledged approach with a passionate community of practitioners and people who swear by it. And no, this isn't just another wellness trend—it's built credibility through real-world applications and testimonials. People are seeing results, feeling more aligned, and sharing their stories. That's how PSYCH-K has become a serious player in the healing game.

The benefits of using PSYCH-K are numerous, particularly for those looking to make lasting changes at a subconscious level. Here are some of the key advantages:

- **Reprogram limiting beliefs:** PSYCH-K helps you identify and transform limiting beliefs that may be holding you back. Whether it's related to self-worth, health, or relationships, you can rewire your subconscious mind to support positive outcomes.

- **Improved mental and emotional health:** PSYCH-K dives straight into your subconscious to kick emotional blocks and mental stress to the curb, often doing a better job than traditional talk therapy. The result? A delightful boost in balance, peace, and all-around well-being!

- **Accelerated personal growth:** Instead of spending years trying to change with conscious effort alone, PSYCH-K speeds up the process. It allows you to break free from old patterns quickly, making personal growth and self-development a reality.

- **Achieving desired outcomes:** Whether it's manifesting your goals or ramping up your career, health, or relationships, PSYCH-K empowers you to align your subconscious beliefs with your conscious desires, making it easier to achieve the results you want.

- **Efficient and easy to use:** PSYCH-K is like the fast food of healing techniques—simple, quick, and no lengthy training required! You can see real changes with just a sprinkle of effort, making it perfect for busy bees.

- **Holistic healing:** PSYCH-K is like a wellness team for your mind, body, and spirit, working together to help you live in peace. It unlocks your inner hero to heal and boosts your overall health!

In summary, PSYCH-K offers a powerful and efficient way to create lasting change by reprogramming your subconscious mind, leading to better mental health, personal growth, and success in achieving your goals.

## *Julie's Story*

Let me tell you about Julie. At just eight years old, she went through some tough times—trauma that left a lasting impact. Instead of shutting down, though, she became obsessed with understanding herself and the world around her. Pre-internet days meant weekends at the library, where she devoured books on psychology, astrology, wellness—you name it. She was drawn to the darker side of human nature, always asking, "Why?"

Years later, Julie realized her intense need to know everything was a response to her trauma. She wanted to see everything coming so she wouldn't get hurt again. This drive set her on a lifelong quest to understand why people respond the way they do and act in ways they do.

Over the next 25+ years, Julie immersed herself in a wide range of subjects—psychology, energy healing, shadow work, meditation, and more. She also tried countless therapies—talk therapy, EMDR, you name it. While these methods helped a bit, none of them felt like the solution.

Julie's trauma showed up as body image issues and disordered eating. From a young age, food became her comfort. She'd sneak cookies when no one was around, and this habit evolved into a lifelong struggle with food, weight, and body image. She tried extreme diets, binged, restricted, and repeated the cycle for years.

At 34, she spent $250 on a hypnotherapy session to control her cravings, only to binge on a family pack of Oreos on the way home. Julie realized she was trying to fix deep, subconscious issues with surface-level tools, which only led to frustration.

Then, she discovered PSYCH-K. In December 2022, Julie stumbled upon it through a social media post and felt an instant connection. By March 2023, she attended a PSYCH-K workshop, and within three days, she made more progress than in years of therapy. She discovered that PSYCH-K worked with her subconscious mind to reprogram her limiting beliefs and outdated patterns. It was fast, effective, and surprisingly fun.

In the months after the workshop, Julie saw real changes. She could finally listen to her body, eat only when hungry, and quit her sugar habit after 25 years. The best part? It didn't require years of effort—just simple, effective steps.

By August 2023, Julie had completed advanced PSYCH-K workshops and continued healing her food-related trauma. The mental space once taken up by food and body issues was now free for her to enjoy her life, explore her creativity, and focus on her future.

Julie's quest isn't over, but in just a few months, she experienced more progress than in 25+ years of other methods. PSYCH-K® became the game-changer she had been searching for—a way to finally break free from the painful cycles and truly transform her life.

## The Science Behind PSYCH-K

Let's dive into the science behind PSYCH-K, shall we? If you've ever wondered if this is more than just another "woo-woo" technique, you're not alone. PSYCH-K may sound out there, but guess what? There's some solid science backing it up. So, let's break it down and see how it all works—no lab coat required.

The research available, while not extensive, shows some promising results that hint at the method's potential to help with changing beliefs. For example, a study by Dr. Jeffrey Fannin used nifty brainwave measuring tech before and after PSYCH-K sessions and found some significant changes in brain function, suggesting that PSYCH-K has a positive impact on mental states (Fannin & Williams, 2011).

## *The Power of Belief*

First, PSYCH-K emphasizes that our beliefs shape our reality. Think of your mind as a movie director, and those beliefs? They're the script. The way you see the world—and your role in it—is colored by what you believe deep down. Studies in cognitive psychology have shown over and over that our beliefs influence everything from our behavior to our perception of stress (McKy, n.d.). When you think, "I can't do this," your brain and body work to prove you right. But here's the kicker: your beliefs can change. Yup, those old thought patterns can be rewritten, and PSYCH-K is one of the tools that can do that.

Neuroplasticity, anyone? That's the fancy term for your brain's ability to change itself. This isn't just motivational poster talk—there's actual science behind it. Research shows that targeted processes can literally rewire your brain (Price & Duman, 2019). PSYCH-K taps into this by using specific techniques to help you shift those limiting beliefs that have been holding you back, reinforcing that change is not only possible but also happening at a neurobiological level.

## *Neuroscience: The Brain-Body Connection*

There's more going on under the hood than you might think. Neurobiological research shows that changing beliefs can alter the brain's pathways—this is what helps PSYCH-K work its magic (Nardone et al., 2017). When you shift a belief, your brain doesn't just passively sit by. Instead, it's actively reconfiguring itself, strengthening the pathways that support this new belief. You're literally rewiring yourself for success.

Studies even suggest that positive belief changes can impact emotional regulation and overall health (Ortner et al., 2017). That means PSYCH-K isn't just a mental exercise; it has real, physiological effects on your body. When you change your mind, your body follows suit.

## Kinesiology and Muscle Testing: The Body's Lie Detector

Now, let's talk muscle testing. Ever tried asking your body a question? No, it's not as weird as it sounds. PSYCH-K uses applied kinesiology—a fancy way of saying your muscles can tell you the truth when your mind tries to lie. Muscle testing serves as a biofeedback tool to tap into the subconscious.

Your subconscious doesn't sugarcoat anything. Through muscle testing, your body gives you a "yes" or "no" answer, depending on whether your subconscious aligns with your conscious beliefs. Imagine it as your body's way of saying, "Nope, we're not buying what you're selling," or, "Yeah, that's the real deal."

Think of muscle testing as a two-way conversation with your body and PSYCH-K as the translator. It helps bring subconscious beliefs to the surface, where they can be understood and shifted. And when you find that your muscles give you a weak response to something you thought was true? That's your cue to dig deeper.

### Muscle Testing in Action: Types and Techniques

Muscle tests come in two types: strength tests and directional tests. Most go for the directional ones for self-testing because they don't wear you out, give you a straight-up answer for yes or no, and are discreet. Give them all a whirl and find your favorite.

Let's break down the different types of muscle tests. Are you ready to test your own body's truth detector? Here's how (Pineda, 2022):

- **Sway test (directional muscle test):** The sway test is as simple as it gets. Stand with your feet shoulder-width apart, take a deep breath, and ask a yes-or-no question. Your body will naturally lean forward for yes and backward for no. It's your body's way of saying, "I'm in alignment with this," or "Nope, not feeling it."

- **Wrist test (directional muscle test):** This one's my personal favorite. Start with your wrist in a neutral position (think comfortably on your lap), and then ask your question. Your wrist will roll outward for yes (think expansion, opening up) and inward for no. It's a subtle but powerful way to check in with your subconscious.

- **Shoulders test (directional muscle test):** In this test, your shoulders will give you the answer. For a yes, they'll open up, expanding at the heart. For a no, they'll slump forward, closing off the heart. It's a small movement, but it can tell you a lot about your inner alignment.

- **Middle finger over index finger (strength muscle test):** For this test, point your index finger and rest the tip of your middle finger on top of your index fingernail. Press your middle finger down while resisting with your index finger. If your index finger stays strong, that's a yes. If it drops, that's a no. This one takes a bit of practice to get just right.

- **Interlocking "O" fingers (strength muscle test):** Create circles with your thumb and index fingers on both hands, interlocking them like a chain. Then, try to pull your fingers apart. If the chain stays strong, that's a yes. If it breaks, that's a no. This test is great for when you need a quick answer.

## *A Step-by-Step Guide to Muscle Testing*

Ready to give muscle testing a try? It's easier than you think, and yes, you can totally do it. Here's your crash course:

1. **Clear your mind:** Take a deep breath and picture all your scattered thoughts coming together like a magnet. Feel yourself stand taller like you're grounding into the earth.

2. **Choose your testing method:** Find a method from above that resonates with you. Say, "Show me a yes," and feel what happens. Then, ask for a "no." Calibration is key here—this is how you and your body start speaking the same language.

3. **Ask a question:** Formulate a clear yes or no question, like, "Is this belief serving me?" Wait for the response—strong for yes, weak for no.

4. **Observe and practice:** If you're feeling unsure, practice makes perfect. Like any skill, muscle testing gets stronger with time.

Feel free to visit the resource page at the end of this book to find some great places to expand your knowledge on muscle testing, along with video tutorials to watch.

PSYCH-K may sound a little out there, but science has its back. From the brain's neuroplasticity to the body's biofeedback system, this technique isn't just talk—it's rooted in research. With a little bit of practice (and maybe some muscle-testing fun), you can start to unlock your potential and release the beliefs holding you back. Ready to see where it takes you?

# Identify Limiting Beliefs: Uncover What's Holding You Back

Okay, let's get real for a second. If you're like most of us, there's a little voice inside your head whispering (or sometimes yelling), "You can't do that," "You're not good enough," or "Why even try?" These are your limiting beliefs talking, and trust me, they are not your friends. But the good news? You don't have to keep listening to them. Using the PSYCH-K approach, you can unmask these sneaky beliefs and be rid of them once and for all. Ready to dive in?

### *Recognizing Patterns of Thought: The First Step to Freedom*

The first step to freeing yourself from limiting beliefs is recognizing the patterns of thought that keep you stuck. It's like realizing that every time you walk into that one room in your house, you stub your toe. After the third or fourth time, you'd probably think, "Wait, maybe I need to do something about this!" It's the same with your thoughts. Let's walk through some important steps:

- **Step 1: Spot the triggers**—Let's start by paying attention to what triggers those emotional reactions you experience daily. Maybe it's when someone criticizes you or when you see someone else achieving something you've always wanted. Whatever it is, there's a belief lurking beneath that emotional response. That's your cue to say, "Aha! There you are!" Write down what triggered you and how you felt in that moment. This is your starting point.

- **Step 2: Reflect on the past**—Now, let's connect the dots. How do these triggers link to your past experiences? Here's a little exercise: Take a moment to think back to a time when you first felt that same emotional reaction. Maybe it's from childhood, maybe it's something more recent. Ask yourself, "When did I first start believing this about myself?" You'll often find that these beliefs are rooted in something long gone, but they've been carried into your present life like a heavy backpack you never put down. Time to unpack it!

- **Step 3: Recognize the Pattern**—Once you've identified a few of these triggers and the beliefs behind them, you'll start to see patterns emerge. Recognizing these patterns is key to initiating change. You might realize that every time something doesn't go perfectly, you tell yourself, "I'm a failure." But the truth is, this belief isn't serving you—it's holding you back. Acknowledging this pattern is the first step to rewriting the script.

## *Practical Exercises for Identification: Let's Get to Work*

Now that you've started identifying those limiting beliefs let's dig even deeper. Let's do some exercises that will help you uncover what's hiding beneath the surface.

## *Journaling Prompt 1: "I Can't Because..."*

Write down something you've been wanting to do but haven't taken action on. Then, finish the sentence: "I can't because…" Don't overthink it—just let whatever comes to mind flow onto the paper. Once you've got a few answers, look for the underlying belief. For example, if you wrote, "I can't start a business because I'm not smart enough," that's a limiting belief right there. Circle it, and let's move on.

_____
_____
_____
_____
_____
_____
_____

## *Journaling Prompt 2: "What's the Worst That Could Happen?"*

Think of a goal or dream you've been putting off. Now ask yourself, "What's the worst that could happen if I actually tried?" Write down your fears. Then, look at them closely. Are these fears based on reality, or are they tied to limiting beliefs? Spoiler alert: They're probably tied to beliefs like "I'll fail" or "I don't deserve success." Time to bust those myths.

_____
_____
_____
_____
_____
_____
_____

*Journaling Prompt 3: "Where Did This Come From?"*

Take one of the limiting beliefs you've identified and ask yourself, "Where did this come from?" Was it something someone told you when you were younger? Was it an experience that made you feel small? Write down the memory that comes to mind. Understanding where a belief originated helps you see that it's not an unchangeable truth—it's just a story you've been telling yourself.

_____
_____
_____
_____
_____
_____

By the end of these exercises, you'll have a clearer picture of the beliefs that have been lurking in the shadows, keeping you from living your best life. And with that awareness, you can start using PSYCH-K techniques to rewrite those beliefs and finally step into your power.

Your future self is waiting—limiting beliefs not invited!

# Guided Sessions: Josh's Story With PSYCH-K

Meet Josh. He's an everyday guy who, after the tragic loss of his wife, found himself struggling to breathe through the fog of grief. He was always the kind of person who would power through things, but this? This was different. Nothing seemed to help—until he stumbled upon PSYCH-K.

At first, Josh was skeptical. It sounded a little too out there for his logical mind. But after feeling stuck for so long, he decided to give it a shot. What he discovered was nothing short of life-changing. PSYCH-K became his way of accessing his subconscious, rewriting the stories that had been holding him back.

Josh didn't just sit in on one or two guided sessions and call it a day. Nope, he integrated PSYCH-K into his daily routine like a well-practiced habit. Every morning, he'd sit with his coffee and perform a simple belief-balance technique. He used this technique to reinforce that he could create peace within himself despite the chaos of his loss. It wasn't complicated or time-consuming—just a few quiet moments to set the tone for his day. Josh found that these few minutes made all the difference. His mornings were no longer filled with dread but with a subtle, reassuring calm.

When life would get messy—like when he couldn't find his car keys and was already running late—Josh used PSYCH-K techniques to keep his stress in check. Instead of spiraling into frustration, he would pause, breathe, and remind himself that he could handle whatever came his way. These moments, though seemingly small, were what helped him maintain a positive mindset. He realized that stress didn't have to control him; he could control how he responded to it.

But the real magic happened in those bigger moments of self-doubt. Like when Josh started dating again. That was tough. The fear of opening up, the guilt of moving forward—PSYCH-K helped him handle all of it. He would use a technique called a "whole-brain posture" to center himself before dates. By simply standing or sitting in a specific way, Josh could align his conscious and subconscious mind, allowing him to be present and confident rather than overwhelmed by the "what ifs."

To foster long-term growth, Josh made sure to incorporate PSYCH-K exercises regularly. On Sunday nights, he'd do a deeper belief-change process to address the bigger things weighing on him—like letting go of guilt or finding joy again. These sessions were his time to check in with himself, to ensure he wasn't just surviving but actively healing and growing.

What Josh learned is that personal growth isn't a one-and-done thing. It's a continual process of showing up for yourself, using tools like PSYCH-K to support your process, and committing to healing daily.

# Reflection and Journaling Exercise: Your Post-Session Moment

After you've worked through a PSYCH-K session, whether it's a quick belief balance or a deeper process, don't rush back into the chaos of life just yet. This is your time to reflect—because reflection isn't just a pause; it's the space where the real growth happens.

Grab a journal, your phone, or even a sticky note. Write down any insights or experiences that came up for you during the session. Maybe you felt a shift, a release, or a new sense of clarity. Putting it into words helps you process what's happening within you.

Think of this journaling exercise as your post-workout stretch. Just like your muscles need time to cool down and integrate the work they've done, your mind and energy need that reflective space too. When you reflect, you hold yourself accountable. You're acknowledging the changes you're making, the beliefs you're challenging, and the progress you're tracking.

Here's a prompt to get you started:

- What limiting belief did I work on today? How do I feel about it now?

- What shifts did I notice in my thoughts, emotions, or body during the session?

- How will I remind myself of this new belief or mindset moving forward?

Tracking your progression and healing is powerful. It's like keeping a map of where you've been so you can see just how far you've come. And trust me, you'll want to look back and celebrate those moments of growth when you realize just how much you've transformed.

Keep journaling, keep reflecting, and keep showing up for yourself. You've got this.

## PSYCH-K Balance Session Form

Here's a template and some sample goal statements to guide you through your PSYCH-K session. This template will show how to integrate muscle testing and balancing techniques into the process of unlocking your body's energy to release trauma.

It will allow you to reflect on your experience after the balancing session.

## Step 1: Set your goal statement

Before we dive into muscle testing, let's get clear on what you want to change or achieve. This is your goal statement—something positive and affirming that you want to embody.

### Example goal statement:

- "I am worthy of love and acceptance, just as I am."

## Step 2: Muscle testing for permission

Now, here's where the magic of your body's energy comes into play. To make sure we're aligned with your subconscious, you'll start by asking for permission to proceed with the balance. The key phrase you'll use is:

- **"Is it safe and appropriate to balance for this goal?"**

You'll need to do a muscle test for a yes or no answer. Remember, your body is always giving you signals—you're just tapping into its natural wisdom.

### Step 3: Pre-balance muscle test

After getting permission, you'll test how your subconscious currently feels about your goal statement. You can use these two examples for the muscle test:

- **Positive statement:** "I am confident in my abilities."
- **Negative statement:** "I am not good enough."

**Muscle test results (pre-balance):** Are you feeling strong or weak when you test these? Jot down your results because we'll revisit this after the balance.

### Step 4: Balance technique – Crossing hands and feet

Here's a simple and effective way to balance your energy:

1. Cross your right hand over your left hand (or the other way around).

2. Cross your right foot over your left foot (or reverse).

3. Sit in this position while you repeat your goal statement (e.g., "I am worthy of love and acceptance, just as I am") in your mind or out loud.

4. Stay like this until you feel a shift—whether it's a change in emotion, a sense of peace, or even a feeling of lightness.

Once you feel that shift, you'll uncross your hands and feet.

**Step 5: Post-balance muscle test**

Now that you've completed the balance, you'll muscle test again:

- **Positive statement:** "I am confident in my abilities."
- **Negative statement:** "I am not good enough."

Test to see if there's a change in how strong or weak you feel with these statements compared to before.

**Step 6: Check if the process is complete**

To make sure the balance is complete, ask your subconscious:

- "Is this process complete?"

Muscle test for a yes or no. If you get a yes, you're done! If you get a no, that's okay—you can simply ask:

- "What do I need to know right now?"

Sometimes, there's more to uncover or another layer to balance, and your subconscious will guide you.

**Step 7: Reflect on how you feel after the balance**

Take a moment to tune in and notice how you feel. You might feel lighter, more peaceful, or just ready to move forward.

- **Example reflection:** "I feel more at peace with myself and confident in my ability to make positive changes."

There has been a page added to the resource page with additional options of balance exercises you can try.

| | | | | |
|---|---|---|---|---|
| Goal Statement | | | | |
| Muscle Test Results (pre-balance) | | | | |
| Balance Technique Used | | | | |
| Muscle Test Results (post-balance) | | | | |
| How I Feel After the Balance | | | | |

## *Sample Goal Statements for PSYCH-K Balance*

This list of sample goal statements to help you feel supported and empowered as you work through your PSYCH-K sessions.

- "I am in alignment with my highest purpose and trust the process ahead."

- "I am enough, just as I am, in every aspect of my life."

- "I am free from the fear of failure and embrace challenges with confidence."

- "I let go of past traumas and embrace my power to heal."

- "I deserve happiness, success, and fulfillment in all areas of my life."

- "I attract healthy, supportive relationships into my life."

- "I trust myself and my decisions completely."

- "I handle stress with ease and remain calm in difficult situations."

- "I feel safe expressing my true self to the world."

- "I release any negative beliefs about money and allow abundance to flow to me."

# Important Considerations for PSYCH-K

When diving into the world of PSYCH-K, there are a few things to keep in mind to make sure you have a safe and effective ride. One major thing to watch out for is those emotional landmines and past traumas that might pop up during sessions. PSYCH-K can stir up some deep emotions or memories you thought were lost in the attic of your mind.

This can hit you out of nowhere, so it's good to know these intense reactions are on the table. Getting a grip on these emotional triggers is like getting your mental warm-up in. For example, if you've faced a significant loss, you might find yourself reliving those heavy feelings of grief or anger. Knowing this can help you approach each session with a mix of caution and an open heart. The aim isn't to shove these emotions under a rug but to let them come up naturally, paving the way for healing and change.

Before diving into any PSYCH-K session, don't forget the safety nets and mental warm-ups. It's all about carving out a calm space where you can just be you—think cozy corners, quiet vibes, and zero distractions. And let's not skip out on getting your head in the game! Know what you want to dig into during the session. Understanding which feelings you're poking at or memories you're sifting through can help keep things on track.

Take a second to ground yourself before you kick things off. A few deep breaths or a quick meditative moment can seriously help to clear your head and settle your body, giving you that much-needed calm when going into emotional territory. Plus, having a buddy around who you trust can be helpful if things get intense. Their support can be like a safety blanket, making it easier to handle those touchy spots in your mind.

In this chapter, we've looked deep into the fascinating world of PSYCH-K, exploring its roots, principles, and practical applications. We've seen how Robert M. Williams' innovative approach in combining elements from neuroscience, biology, and mind-body integration aims to transform limiting beliefs and reprogram the subconscious mind for personal growth. By utilizing techniques like whole-brain integration and muscle testing, individuals can uncover and shift deep-seated belief patterns that shape their everyday experiences.

Whether you're struggling with self-esteem, anxiety, or health issues, PSYCH-K offers a holistic and gentle method to address these challenges. Its potential extends beyond personal development, touching aspects of physical health and spiritual connectedness as well. With its emphasis on creating a safe and balanced environment, PSYCH-K ensures you can pursue meaningful change without reliving past traumas. As you consider integrating PSYCH-K into your life, remember that patience and consistency are key to unlocking its full benefits, leading you toward a more empowered and balanced self.

Let's move into the next chapter and discover the healing powers of Reiki.

# Chapter 5:
# The Healing World of Reiki

Harnessing Reiki for healing can sound like learning to ride a magical, invisible bike powered by good energy. It's all about tapping into universal life energy and channeling it to where it's needed most. Imagine you're a human wi-fi router, spreading high-speed positive vibes. But instead of connecting devices, you're helping to balance your own or energy fields. In this chapter, we'll walk through the ins and outs of Reiki, providing explanations and sharing stories that illustrate its power in healing trauma and ramping up self-worth.

Ready for some real-world magic? In this chapter, you'll discover the ethical principles that guide practitioners and ensure sessions are safe, respectful, and nurturing. Get comfortable and prepare to explore the soothing, restorative power of Reiki!

## An Overview of Reiki

Imagine you're living in early 20th-century Japan, a time filled with mystique and tradition. Enter Mikao Usui, a man on a quest for spiritual enlightenment who ultimately gifts the world Reiki, a holistic healing technique that has touched countless lives since its inception. Developed around the 1920s, Reiki combines profound simplicity with deep spiritual insights, creating a method accessible to all who seek its benefits. Usui's unique approach distilled many pre-existing concepts into one straightforward system, making it a revolutionary healing modality (*What Is the History of Reiki?*, 2014). So, let's explore this fascinating practice together and see how it can help heal stored trauma.

## The Ethical Framework

To unveil Reiki's fundamentals, it's important to recognize the ethical framework that underpins practice. Reiki practitioners abide by specific guidelines aimed at fostering an atmosphere of compassion and respect. This begins with the principles of Reiki, encapsulated in the Five Precepts or Gokai, which emphasize:

- gratitude
- integrity
- humility
- kindness
- calmness

It is fundamental that these values guide every session, ensuring a safe and nurturing environment for both the practitioner and recipient.

## How Reiki Works

So, how does Reiki work its magic? In essence, it's about channeling universal life energy from the practitioner to the recipient. Imagine the practitioner as a conduit, tapping into a vast reservoir of positive energy and gently directing it where it's needed most.

This process helps balance the body's energy fields, facilitating emotional release and restoring equilibrium. The beauty of Reiki lies in its non-invasive nature. There are no needles, potions, or elaborate rituals involved, just the gentle laying on of hands—sometimes even without physical contact—which allows the energy to flow and do its work.

So why should you consider Reiki, especially if you're dealing with trauma? The practice promotes deep relaxation, which is vital for anyone struggling with emotional turmoil. When the body relaxes, it enters a state where healing can occur more naturally and effortlessly. By easing tension and fostering inner peace, Reiki paves the way for emotional release and self-awareness, crucial steps in healing from trauma.

## Common Reiki Myths Debunked

You might be wondering, "Isn't this just a placebo?" or "Is Reiki some sort of religion?" These are common misconceptions that need debunking.

- **Reiki is a religion:** Many people think Reiki is like joining a secret religious club—sacred robes, secret handshakes, and maybe even a magic wand! But no! Reiki is actually a spiritual healing practice open to everyone, regardless of their belief system. It's like a buffet of good energy where anyone can grab a plate!

- **Reiki is just a placebo:** Some think that Reiki is just a fancy placebo. Sure, a sprinkle of faith might jazz it up, but plenty of people, even the biggest skeptics—those who roll their eyes more than they roll out their yoga mats—report feeling way less stressed and achy after a good Reiki session and yes there is science to back it up

(Demir Doğan, 2018)! Who knew that mystical energy could work wonders, even on the doubtful?

- **Reiki is only effective in person:** With the rise of virtual services, some think Reiki only works if you're in the same room as if it's a high-tech hide-and-seek game. But Reiki practitioners can channel energy from afar, proving that you don't need to be shoulder-to-shoulder to experience a healing touch—no teleportation required!

- **Reiki is difficult to learn:** Some think that learning Reiki requires years of training. In fact, Reiki is like the universal remote of wellness—accessible to anyone who's willing to learn. With the proper instruction, anyone can channel their inner healing powers and practice Reiki.

- **Reiki is a new age fad:** Although Reiki has gained popularity in recent years—probably thanks to the stress levels of modern life—it's not exactly a new kid on the block. As we discussed, it came to light in the early 20th century. Its principles are deeply rooted in the concept of universal life energy, a notion that various cultures have been nodding at for a very long time.

In addressing these misconceptions and deepening our understanding of the practice, it becomes clear that Reiki can be an invaluable part of our healing toolkit, like a Swiss Army knife for the spirit. It operates on the principle that our bodies and minds are interconnected, much like a web of energy. When trauma disrupts this web, Reiki helps mend it by restoring balance and harmony, reminding us that simplicity can pack a punch and effectiveness doesn't need to wear a lab coat.

# Benefits of Reiki Healing

Reiki offers so many benefits, especially when it comes to taking care of stored trauma and bolstering self-worth. You might wonder how this practice manages to wield such power. Let's dive into some personal tales and simple explanations to uncover the diverse advantages of Reiki.

## *Releasing Suppressed Emotions*

First, one of the most profound benefits of Reiki lies in its ability to release suppressed emotions. Picture yourself like a soda bottle that's been shaken up too many times. That fizzy pressure inside is your unresolved emotions waiting to explode. Reiki acts like a slow, gentle twist of the cap, letting all that pent-up energy escape without chaos. During a session, you might find yourself feeling unexpectedly emotional. This isn't just random; it's the process of buried feelings coming to light and finally being acknowledged. As these emotions surface, you may experience an incredible sense of relief and mental clarity. It's similar to clearing out a cluttered attic—you suddenly have space for fresh air and new perspectives. Let's look at a story to illustrate this a little more closely.

### *Elle's Journey With Reiki*

Elle had always felt emotionally heavy, the kind of weighed down that was impossible to see. It started in her childhood when her father left, and no one ever talked about it. The silence surrounding his absence felt like a storm waiting to break, but the storm never came—it just lingered, causing fear and uncertainty to become Elle's constant companions. As she grew older, she found herself in relationships that echoed her early experiences. Men who promised stability but left her feeling even more adrift when they inevitably walked away.

She tried to move on, throwing herself into work, friendships, and things to keep her busy, but something always felt off. It was as if all the unresolved emotions were bottled up inside her, fizzing and building pressure with nowhere to go. Regardless of how hard she tried to ignore it, the fear of abandonment lingered in the background, shaping her decisions and keeping her on edge.

One day, a close coworker suggested Reiki. Elle had many questions. How could something as simple as energy healing help her when years of talking, journaling, and self-reflection hadn't? But something about the idea intrigued her, so she decided to give it a try.

During her first Reiki session, Elle didn't know what to expect. The room was peaceful, with soft music playing in the background. As the Reiki practitioner gently placed their hands just above Elle's body, she felt an unfamiliar sensation—like a warm, soothing space was slowly untangling knots inside her.

And then, out of nowhere, Elle felt tears welling up in her eyes. She wasn't sure why she was crying; nothing specific came to mind. But it wasn't the same kind of overwhelming sobbing she'd experienced during difficult moments in her past. This felt different—gentler, like a slow, controlled release of something deep inside her. Her soda bottle cap had been twisted ever so slightly, letting out the pressure without the explosion she had feared for so long.

As the session continued, memories began to surface. Not the sharp, painful ones she'd revisited in therapy, but the small, forgotten moments that had shaped her fears. The time her father missed her birthday. The way her ex-boyfriend had casually mentioned moving to another city without even discussing it with her. Each memory floated to the surface, was acknowledged, but then, more importantly—safely released.

By the end of the session, Elle felt lighter—not just physically, but emotionally. It was as if she had cleared out a cluttered closet that had been stuffed full of old, forgotten things. Now, there was room for light, new perspectives, and a sense of calm she hadn't known in years.

Reiki didn't solve all of Elle's problems that day, but it gave her something she hadn't realized she was missing: space. Space to breathe, reflect, and finally start healing from the inside out.

## *Physical Healing*

Beyond emotional relief, Reiki puts the spotlight on physical healing. Let's say you continue to wake up with a nagging backache that seems to love haunting you during stressful periods. Now think about lying down for a Reiki session where the practitioner's hands hover gently over your pain points. As minutes tick by, you feel warmth and a tingling sensation. By the end of the session, the ache has dulled or even vanished. How is this possible? Reiki essentially channels energy into areas of stagnation, promoting blood flow and reducing inflammation. Studies suggest that it lowers stress hormones like cortisol, which are often culprits in chronic pain and anxiety (*The Benefits of Reiki*, 2024). When cortisol levels drop, your body shifts from a state of stress to one of healing, supporting overall recovery. Again, let's look at a relatable story to bring this all together.

## *Callie's Neck Pain*

Callie had been dealing with neck pain for as long as she could remember. It seemed to get worse during the busiest times at work—deadlines looming, meetings piling up, and her stress levels climbing higher and higher. She had tried to ignore it for years, thinking it was just something she had to live with. Massage therapy helped, but only for a few days. Medications weren't an option for her since she was allergic to most, so she sought out holistic solutions.

That's when her naturopath recommended Reiki. Callie was willing to give anything a try if it meant finding some pain relief.

Walking into the Reiki session, Callie felt both curious and apprehensive. She instantly loved walking into the room because it was calming, filled with soft light and the soothing scent of essential oils. The practitioner explained that during the session, they would focus on channeling energy to areas of tension and stagnation, like her neck. Callie lay down on the table, closing her eyes as the session began.

The practitioner's hands hovered gently over Callie's neck, and for the first few minutes, she wasn't sure if anything was happening. Slowly, she began to notice warmth spreading across her neck and shoulders. A gentle tingling sensation followed as if the tension that had been locked in her muscles was starting to fade away.

As the session continued, Callie found herself slipping into a deep state of relaxation. The usual tightness in her neck began to ease, and by the time the session ended, she felt like she had just woken up from the most restful sleep of her life. The pain that had haunted her for years had dulled to a manageable twinge.

Over the next few days, Callie noticed something remarkable. The pain didn't come roaring back like it usually did after a massage. Instead, she felt a lingering sense of calm, as if her body had finally started to heal itself. She decided to incorporate Reiki into her regular life, scheduling sessions every few weeks.

Callie also began practicing what she called "mini Reiki moments" during her workday. When the stress started building up, she would close her eyes, take a few deep breaths, and visualize the warmth and healing energy from her Reiki sessions flowing through her neck and shoulders. It wasn't a cure-all, but it helped her manage the stress before it could manifest as physical pain.

Over time, Callie realized that Reiki was doing more than just helping with her neck pain. She felt less anxious, more centered, and better equipped to handle the demands of her job. The combination of regular Reiki sessions and her daily mindfulness practice had shifted her body from a constant state of stress to one of healing.

## *Reiki and Relaxation*

Speaking of stress, we can't overlook how superbly Reiki fosters relaxation. Modern life is a whirlwind of never-ending to-do lists and responsibilities. This lifestyle leads to heightened cortisol levels, contributing to both physical ailments and emotional turbulence. When you settle into a Reiki session, it's like hitting the pause button on life. The act of lying still, with calming music playing, encourages your nervous system to enter a parasympathetic state. This is the body's rest-and-digest mode, opposite to fight-or-flight. In this state, your body can repair itself, digest food more efficiently, and build immunity. Over time, regular Reiki sessions can create a habit of relaxation and greatly diminish the adverse effects of chronic stress and trauma.

Reiki doesn't just stop at healing the body and mind; it also nurtures self-awareness and empowerment. Think of yourself standing in front of a foggy mirror every morning—not exactly a riveting start, right? It's frustrating not seeing yourself clearly, like trying to find your keys in a messy room. Reiki acts like a determined hand wiping away the mist. Each session helps you connect deeply with your inner self, kind of like a GPS recalculating your route when you've taken a wrong turn.

A friend of mine once said that after her third Reiki session, she felt as if she had finally come face-to-face with her true self, like a selfie without the filter. She noticed a newfound sense of worth that encouraged her to set healthier boundaries and chase after activities that actually sparked joy—because life's too short for anything less than that. Self-awareness blossoms into self-worth, and Reiki provides the fertile ground for this growth, much like a garden—minus the weeding.

Reiki offers a holistic approach to healing that hits multiple targets simultaneously. It addresses the emotional backlog by surfacing and releasing suppressed feelings—like cleaning out your junk drawer, but way more cathartic. This leads to improved mental health and clarity. Its physical benefits are equally compelling, aiding in pain alleviation, reducing stress, and fostering overall bodily recovery. Promoting deep relaxation and lowering cortisol levels helps mitigate the harmful effects of chronic stress and trauma—making sure you can tackle life's messiness with calm energy. Remember, the practice builds self-awareness and empowers you, paving the way for improved self-worth and personal fulfillment—because who doesn't want to be the best version of themselves?

## Considerations When Practicing Reiki

There are several key points to consider when making your Reiki sessions safe, effective, and truly transformative.

First, finding a qualified Reiki practitioner is crucial. You wouldn't trust just anyone to cut your hair, right? The same applies here—a skilled practitioner guarantees that you have a safe and productive healing experience. Look for someone certified by reputable organizations or has good reviews from previous clients. Meeting them beforehand helps you gauge their energy and approach, which should resonate with you. Trust your gut; if something feels off, continue your search until you find someone who makes you feel completely comfortable.

Once you've found the right practitioner, let's talk about adding self-Reiki techniques to your healing arsenal. Imagine having the ability to channel calming, balancing energies anytime you need! It's like having a personal, pocket-sized wellness coach. Learning simple hand placements and techniques allows you to give yourself mini Reiki sessions.

Start by placing your hands over your heart and taking deep breaths. This can be done first thing in the morning or before bed to set a peaceful tone for your day or night. Self-Reiki empowers you, putting the power of healing directly into your own hands, quite literally.

Creating a soothing environment for your Reiki practice is another necessary step. Your surroundings significantly influence the effectiveness of your healing process. Think of it as setting the stage for a beautiful performance—ambient lighting, soft music, and perhaps some aromatic candles can work wonders. Your space should feel like a sanctuary, a place where you can retreat from the hustle and bustle of daily life. Even something as simple as de-cluttering a room can make a big difference. When your physical space is calm and inviting, your mind can relax more easily, making it simpler to tap into the healing energies.

It's also important to set realistic expectations. Sometimes, we jump into things with sky-high hopes, only to crash land when reality hits. With Reiki, it's important to understand that everyone's experience is unique. One person might feel immediate emotional release, while another may experience subtle shifts over time. Don't stress if you don't see instant results; instead, welcome the process. Reiki isn't a magic pill but a gentle tool that supports your healing in its own sweet time. Communicating these realistic expectations with your practitioner can also help reduce any anxiety you may have, paving the way for a more fulfilling experience.

So, there you have it: A starter kit for handling your Reiki process effectively and safely. Finding a qualified practitioner sets the foundation, self-Reiki techniques integrate healing into your daily life, creating a calm space enhances the process, and managing expectations keeps you grounded and open. Each of these steps contributes to a richer, more balanced healing.

## James' Step By Step Reiki Session

James is a hardworking man who's been dealing with severe back pain and anxiety ever since a work-related accident five years ago. He's tried different therapies, but nothing seems to provide lasting relief. A few people have recommended Reiki, and while

James is hesitant, he decides to give it a shot. Here's how James (and you) can prepare for his Reiki session and make the most of it.

## *Step 1: Pre-Session Preparation*

- **Arrive relaxed:** James's first step is to arrive at his session as relaxed as possible. He knows that showing up stressed out would make it harder for him to receive the full benefits. On the way to his session, James listens to his favorite chill-out playlist. Once he parks, he spends a few minutes doing some deep breathing exercises to calm his mind.

- **Use mindfulness techniques:** James also incorporates mindfulness to center himself. He sits quietly, focusing on his breath, allowing any lingering anxiety to fade away. This simple act helps align his energy, making him more receptive to Reiki's healing power. It's like tuning an instrument before a concert; James is getting energetically tuned for his session.

## *Step 2: During the Session*

- **Set your intentions:** When James arrives, the Reiki practitioner asks him about his goals for the session. James explains that he's been struggling with back pain and anxiety. The practitioner listens carefully and assures him that Reiki can help channel healing energy to these areas of concern.

- **Relax and be present:** James then lies down on the massage table, fully clothed, with his shoes off. The room is serene, with soothing music and the calming scent of lavender in the air. As the session begins, James feels the practitioner's hands hovering over his back and shoulders. Slowly, he starts to notice a gentle warmth and a tingling sensation, like sunlight bathing his skin. He giggles, and guess what? This is normal. No judgment, you do you!

Throughout the session, James makes an effort to stay present. Whenever his mind begins to wander, he brings his focus back to his breath or to the sensations he's feeling. This simple mindfulness helps deepen his experience, allowing the Reiki energy to flow more freely.

## *Step 3: Post-Session Integration*

- **Journaling for reflection:** After the session, James feels lighter and more at ease, but he knows this is only the beginning. To help integrate the healing, once home, he takes a few moments to journal. He writes about the warmth he felt during the session and how his back pain seemed to melt away. He isn't shy about noting his giggle outburst and his fear of flatulence. Remember, this is your journal; feel free to write anything. This reflective practice helps solidify the benefits, giving his experiences a home rather than letting them drift away.

- **Meditation to seal the good energy:** James also sets aside time for a short meditation. Just five to ten minutes of quiet reflection helps him ground the energetic shifts from the Reiki session. He notices that his meditation feels deeper, almost as if his energy field has been rebalanced and renewed. It is no secret that James struggles with this in the beginning. First, he is not used to allowing him time for himself. After practicing, he finds he actually really enjoys it.

- **Complementary practices:** James adds some complementary practices to his routine. When he lets the dog out, he spends a few minutes each morning standing barefoot on the grass, grounding his energy through earthing. When he read about this one, he knew he would love it. He also makes sure to drink plenty of water post-session to keep his energy flowing smoothly. Beyond that, he incorporates deep rest into his day—not just lounging in front of the TV, but real, unplugged rest, like lying down with a weighted blanket and letting his nervous system soak in the tranquility. James had to let go of the stigma that men don't need this type of self-care, and it has changed his healing completely.

## *Step 4: Enhancing the Experience*

- **Spiritual practices:** As the weeks progress, James decides to give other spiritual practices a try to amplify the benefits of Reiki. Once a week, writing down three things he's grateful for. This simple act of focusing on gratitude helps him raise his vibration, reinforcing the positive energy from Reiki and encouraging emotional healing. This added layer of spiritual connection deepens his experience, helping him feel more connected to himself and his healing process.

By following these practical steps, James not only finds relief from his back pain and anxiety but also begins to incorporate Reiki into his regular life. His sessions become part of his overall wellness routine, bringing him a sense of balance and peace he hadn't felt in years.

Reiki is an ongoing process rather than a one-off event. Scheduling regular sessions can help you maintain those heightened energy levels and continue peeling away layers of stored trauma. Think of it as your spiritual gym membership. Just like consistent physical exercise yields better results, regular Reiki sessions deepen your healing and change.

# Can I Do Reiki On Myself?

So, you're wondering if you can do Reiki on yourself? Absolutely! Sure, you won't be practicing it as deeply as a seasoned Reiki master, but let's be real—you've got hands, you've got energy, and you're ready to roll. With a bit of consistency, you can totally make Reiki a part of your self-care routine. Here's how to get started:

- **Step 1: Get comfortable:** First, find a comfy spot. Seriously, don't overthink this part. Sit, stand, lie down, do whatever feels right. Maybe you're a cross-legged-on-a-meditation-cushion kind of person, or perhaps you're all about lying down with your feet propped up like royalty. Either way, make sure your body's supported. You don't want to be mid-Reiki and realize your leg's gone numb. Find that sweet spot where you're relaxed but not at risk of falling asleep (unless that's your goal).

- **Step 2: Give yourself a high five for showing up:** Okay, now that you're comfy, let's take a moment to celebrate something important—you're actually doing this! You've set aside time to practice Reiki on yourself, and that deserves some recognition. Life's crazy, and carving out time for self-care isn't always easy, so pat yourself on the back. Just showing up for yourself is a big deal.

- **Step 3: Breathe (no, really, just breathe):** Time to breathe. Yes, it sounds simple, but have you checked in with your breath lately? Let's drop those shoulders away from your ears, unclench that jaw, and take a deep breath. Feel your body start to loosen up. Imagine that breath traveling to all those tense spots—whether it's your tight shoulders, achy lower back, or the part of you that's carrying the weight of the world. Keep breathing until you feel your body go, "Ahhh, that's better."

- **Step 4: Channel your inner Reiki philosopher:** Now, let's get all Zen for a moment. Remember those cool principles Mikao Usui initiated. These are like your Reiki "rules to live by," except way more chill than actual rules. You can recite these, reflect on them, or just let them hang out in the back of your mind. They're like your Reiki cheat sheet for life. They go like this:

    o  Just for today, don't get angry (easier said than done, right?).

    o  Don't worry (you've got this).

    o  Be grateful (even for that weird, squeaky noise your car makes).

    o  Work diligently (but don't overdo it).

    o  Be kind to yourself and others (especially when someone cuts you off in traffic).

- **Step 5: Call in the calvary (optional but fun):** Feeling a little extra spiritual today? You can totally call in your guides, angels, or that wise, all-knowing voice that lives in your head (you know the one). Imagine inviting them into your session, like, "Hey, Reiki masters, come on in and sprinkle some good energy on this!" Whether you sense their presence or not, just trust that you've got some good intentions supporting you. If nothing else, it makes the session feel a little more positive.

- **Step 6: Get handsy (in a good way):** Here's where the real action happens. You don't need to be a Reiki master to give yourself some healing. Just place your hands on whatever part of your body needs a little love. Maybe it's your heart, your head, your sore back—wherever you feel called. Imagine that warm, glowing energy flowing from your hands into that area, like you're charging your own internal battery. It's like giving yourself a calm with the universe's energy.

- **Step 7: Say thanks and wrap it up:** When you're done, take a moment to say thanks—to yourself, to the energy, to the journey that brought you here. Give yourself a little gratitude for showing up and doing the work. Trust that the life force has been balanced in all the right ways, and release the session with a gentle sense of closure. You've done it. You've just given yourself some well-deserved Reiki love.

Feel free to follow these sessions with the same steps as you would if you visited a practitioner.

# Final Thoughts

As you move forward, remember that Reiki is a gentle tool in your healing toolkit, not an instant fix. Welcome it with an open heart and enjoy the time rather than seeking immediate results. It blends beautifully with other treatments like meditation and therapy, creating a holistic approach to well-being.

So why not give it a shot? With each session, you might find yourself peeling away those emotional layers and stepping closer to a more balanced, serene you. Keep exploring, stay curious, and let Reiki guide you toward deeper healing and self-discovery. Let's continue on to the next chapter, where we will discuss the amazing benefits of somatic healing practices.

## Chapter 6:
# Somatic Experiences

Exploring somatic practices offers a gateway to holistic well-being. Imagine a practice where you get to wiggle, jiggle, and sway your body in ways that feel as natural as breathing and as expressive as a passionate dance-off on your living room floor. Somatic practices help you forge a deep connection with your physical self, uncovering those pesky traumas and emotions that have taken up residence in your muscles and tissues—think of it as a garage sale for your psyche!

Are you ready to wade into the delightful pool of all the types of somatic healing practices, each splashing about with its own methods for helping you release that emotional baggage and trauma that your body is all too happy to part with? You'll discover the principles behind these practices and how they can boost your health and balance.

## What Is Somatic Healing?

Somatic healing is a fascinating and transformative practice that emphasizes your body's natural ability to heal from trauma and release pent-up emotions. At its core, somatic healing operates on the principle that our bodies are not just passive vessels but active participants in our emotional and psychological well-being. This approach recognizes that trauma isn't solely stored in the mind; it often also finds a home in our physical bodies.

Imagine experiencing a stressful situation where your muscles tighten, your heart races, and you feel a knot in your stomach. These are not merely mental reactions but physical expressions of stress and trauma. Over time, if these feelings aren't addressed, they can become ingrained in your muscles and tissues. Somatic healing aims to address these physical manifestations, helping you release these stored emotions and traumas.

One of the foundational beliefs in somatic healing is that trauma can reside in your body long after the initial event has passed. Research shows us that this kind of stored trauma can disrupt your overall health, manifesting as chronic pain, tension, or even more severe ailments like fibromyalgia or autoimmune disorders (Harvard Health Publishing, 2019). When we understand the connection between trauma and physical health, somatic healing provides a pathway for holistic recovery.

Techniques used in somatic healing often involve various forms of physical movement. These movements help to shift energy through and out of your body, releasing the stored tension and emotional baggage. Think of this as internal housekeeping, sweeping away the cobwebs and stagnant energy that have taken up residence in your muscles and tissues. The goal is to get this energy flowing smoothly again, promoting a sense of freedom and lightness both physically and emotionally.

## Types of Somatic Therapies

Somatic therapy is getting the spotlight lately, as people are hitting the walls of traditional talk therapy, and TikTok is all about the buzz. But let's be real: Diving into the jargon jungle of different somatic therapies can feel like trying to untangle a pair of earbuds!

Let's take a closer look at the five kinds of somatic therapy approaches: Somatic Experiencing (SE), Accelerated

Experiential Dynamic Psychotherapy (AEDP), Sensorimotor Psychotherapy, Eye movement desensitization and reprocessing (EMDR), and Gestalt.

Here's a breakdown of them (*5 Kinds of Somatic Therapy*, 2022):

## *Somatic Experiencing (SE): Shaking Off the Stress*

Imagine you're a deer. You've just dodged a predator, and now you're safely grazing again. What do you do to shake off that stress? You literally shake it off! Humans, on the other hand, tend to hold onto stress. Somatic Experiencing is like giving yourself permission to do what that deer does: Shake, tremble, and release all that pent-up tension after a tough experience. You don't even need to relive the trauma in detail; instead, you learn to go back and forth between feeling charged and calm. Think of it as a way to "reset" your nervous system, one small step (or shake) at a time.

### The Pendulation Exercise

Here's a simple Somatic Experiencing (SE) exercise that helps you release stored tension in your body. This exercise focuses on "pendulation," a key concept in SE, where you move between states of discomfort and calmness to help your nervous system discharge stress.

**Purpose:** This exercise is designed to help you release stored tension in your body by gently moving between states of activation (where you feel tension or discomfort) and states of calmness or ease. It helps your nervous system naturally regulate and discharge stress without overwhelming yourself.

*Instructions:*

1. **Get cozy:** Choose a comfortable, quiet spot where you feel safe and can relax. Sit or lie down in a position that feels supportive to your body. Take a few deep breaths to settle into the present moment.

2. **Notice your body:** Begin by gently scanning your body from head to toe. Pay attention to any areas where you feel tension, discomfort, or a sense of activation. It could be tightness in your neck, a knot in your stomach, or even a sense of restlessness. Don't try to fix or change it—just notice and observe.

3. **Focus on the sensation:** Choose one area of tension or discomfort to focus on. Bring your awareness to that sensation and notice what it feels like. Is it sharp, dull, tight, or heavy? How big or small is it? Stay curious and explore it with gentle attention.

4. **Pendulate to calmness:** Now, shift your focus away from the tension and find a place in your body that feels neutral or calm. It could be your hands, feet, or anywhere that feels at ease. Take a few moments to really feel that calmness or neutral sensation in your body. Allow yourself to rest in this state for a bit.

5. **Go back and forth:** Gently move your attention back to the area of tension or discomfort. Spend a few seconds noticing it, then shift your focus back to the area of calmness or ease. Continue this back-and-forth movement—this "pendulation"—between the uncomfortable and calm sensations in your body. Do

this at your own pace, going back to the calm sensation whenever you feel the need.

6. **Release the tension:** After several rounds of pendulation, notice if the area of tension has shifted or softened. You may feel the discomfort start to dissolve or move through your body. If it feels right, you can also gently shake your hands, feet, or body to help release any remaining tension, similar to how animals shake off stress after a threat.

7. **Rest and Reflect:** After you've completed the exercise, take a few moments to rest. Reflect on how your body feels now compared to when you started. Answer the following:

    A. Do you notice any changes in your physical or emotional state?

_____
_____
_____
_____
_____
_____

*Why This Helps*

The pendulation exercise teaches your body how to move between states of activation and relaxation. This helps your nervous system learn to regulate itself more effectively. By gently touching into uncomfortable sensations and then retreating to calmness, you gradually release stored tension without overwhelming your system.

This is a great exercise to do whenever you feel stressed, anxious, or like you're holding onto something heavy in your body. It's about finding balance and helping your body gently let go of what no longer serves you. It can be a great way to begin or end your day.

## *Sensorimotor Psychotherapy: Your Body Remembers*

Let's take a trip down memory lane, not in your head, but in your body. Ever notice how certain postures or movements bring up old feelings? Sensorimotor Psychotherapy is all about tuning into those body memories. Maybe when you slouch, it takes you back to feeling unworthy or unloved. This therapy helps you become aware of how your body is holding onto old patterns and supports you in changing those movements. Imagine learning to stand tall, not just physically but emotionally too, as you rewrite those old stories stored in your muscles.

### The Body Posture Awareness Exercise

Here's a simple exercise inspired by Sensorimotor Psychotherapy that helps you tune into how your body holds onto old emotions and patterns. This exercise encourages awareness of your posture and movements, which are often connected to past experiences.

**Purpose:** This exercise helps you become aware of how your body stores emotional experiences and how changing your posture can impact your emotional state.

*Instructions:*

1. **Find a peaceful spot:** Sit or stand comfortably in a quiet space where you won't be disturbed for a few minutes. Take a few deep breaths to settle in.

2. **Tune into your body:** Start by noticing how your body feels in this moment. Are you tense anywhere? Are you slouching? Is there any discomfort or stiffness? Don't judge what you find; just observe. Take a mental note of your overall posture and physical sensations.

3. **Explore your posture:** Think of a time when you felt small, unimportant, or defeated. Gently allow your body to adopt the posture you naturally take on in that emotional state. Maybe you find your shoulders slumping forward, your head hanging low, or your chest caving in. Notice how your body shapes itself based on this memory or feeling.

4. **Feel the emotion:** As you hold this posture, notice what emotions arise. How does your body feel in this position? Does it feel familiar? Do you feel heavy, sad, or perhaps frustrated? Stay with these sensations for a moment, just observing without trying to change anything.

5. **Shift your posture:** Now, slowly start to change your posture. Sit or stand up straight, lift your head, roll your shoulders back, and open up your chest. Imagine

embodying a sense of confidence, worthiness, or calm. How does this new posture feel? Do you notice any changes in your emotional state? Stay in this position for a few deep breaths, allowing yourself to fully experience the shift.

6. **Reflect:** After a few minutes, gently return to a neutral position and take a moment to reflect on what you experienced. Answer the following questions:

    o How did your emotions shift as you changed

- your posture?

_____
_____
_____
_____
_____
_____

- Did any memories or thoughts arise?

_____
_____
_____
_____
_____
_____

### *Why This Helps*

Sensorimotor Psychotherapy highlights the body-emotion tango. When you tune into your usual stances and try out some fresh moves, you can start shaking off those old patterns clinging to your muscles and move into new emotional rhythms.

Whenever you're in a rut or just want to see how your body is holding stress like a squirrel with acorns, give this exercise a whirl. It's an easy-peasy way to tap into your body's sage advice and make tiny tweaks that can lead to enormous boosts in your emotional health.

## *Accelerated Experiential Dynamic Psychotherapy (AEDP): Healing Through Connection*

Ever had a moment where you felt an emotion so intensely but couldn't share it with anyone? AEDP therapists want to be there for you in those moments. They believe that emotions like grief, joy, and fear are meant to guide us, but when we feel them alone, it's like carrying a heavy suitcase all by ourselves. In AEDP, the therapist is right there with you, helping you unpack that suitcase. They don't just sit back; they engage with you, share their own feelings, and help you feel safe enough to dive into those emotions together. It's all about connection, so you don't have to heal alone.

### *The Core Emotion Connection Exercise*

Here's a simple exercise inspired by Accelerated Experiential Dynamic Psychotherapy (AEDP) that focuses on connecting with your core emotions in a safe and supportive way. This exercise emphasizes self-compassion and the healing power of feeling your emotions while staying connected to yourself.

**Purpose:** This exercise helps you connect with and process your core emotions (such as sadness, grief, happiness, fear, and anger) in a safe and nurturing way, allowing for emotional healing and growth. It also emphasizes creating a compassionate connection with yourself, which is central to AEDP.

*Instructions:*

1. **Create a safe and supportive environment:** Find a peaceful space to sit or lie comfortably. Make sure you feel safe and supported. You might want a blanket or

something that makes you feel cozy. Take a few deep breaths to ground yourself in the present moment.

2. **Invite self-compassion:** Place your hands on your heart or another part of your body that feels soothing, like your stomach or shoulders. Take a few moments to send yourself some gentle compassion. You might silently say to yourself, "It's okay to feel what I'm feeling," or "I'm here for myself."

3. **Identify a core emotion:** Think of a recent experience that brought up a strong emotion for you. It could be something that made you feel upset, mad, ungrateful, or scared. Don't dive too deep into the story—just focus on the emotion the experience stirred up. Allow that emotion to gently surface.

4. **Feel the emotion in your body:** Where do you feel this emotion in your body? Is it a heaviness in your chest, tightness in your throat, warmth in your belly? Take a few moments to really feel that emotion in your body without trying to push it away. Just allow it to be there, noticing its sensations and qualities.

5. **Stay present with the emotion:** Instead of trying to "fix" or change the emotion, simply stay present with it. Imagine you're sitting with a friend who's feeling this emotion, offering them comfort just by being there. You're doing the same for yourself. If the emotion feels overwhelming, remind yourself that it's okay to take small steps. You can always return to this exercise later if needed.

6. **Acknowledge the emotion's purpose:** Ask yourself, "What is this emotion trying to tell me?" Emotions are messengers—they're trying to guide you toward something. Maybe sadness is telling you that you need

rest, or anger is urging you to set a boundary. Gently listen to what the emotion is communicating without judgment.

7. **Feel the emotion shift:** As you stay with the emotion and allow it to be fully felt, notice if it begins to shift. It might soften, intensify, or change into something else. Be curious about this shift, and continue offering yourself compassion as the emotion moves through you.

8. **Connect with a positive emotion:** After spending some time with the core emotion, gently shift your focus to a positive emotion—perhaps a moment of joy, love, or gratitude. Notice how this positive emotion feels in your body. Allow it to expand and fill your entire being, creating a sense of warmth and safety.

9. **Reflect on the experience:** Take a few moments to reflect on the experience. Answer the following:

    o How did it feel to stay present with your emotion?

    _____
    _____
    _____
    _____
    _____

    o Did you notice any shifts or changes?

    _____
    _____
    _____

_____
_____

       o  How does your body feel now compared to when you started?

_____
_____
_____
_____

***Why This Helps***

AEDP focuses on the power of connecting with core emotions in a safe, supportive environment. This exercise is like a personal cheerleader, encouraging you to welcome self-compassion, hang out with your emotions, and let them lead you on a healing quest.

When you give your feelings a full-fledged VIP experience and mingle with the positive energy, you open the door to emotional change. Feel free to hit replay on this exercise whenever your emotions need a good processing session, allowing you to reconnect with yourself in the coziest way possible. It's all about nurturing a loving relationship with your feelings, one delightful step at a time.

## *Eye Movement Desensitization and Reprocessing (EMDR): Rewiring Your Brain*

This one sounds a bit sci-fi at first, but it's pretty straightforward. Think of EMDR as giving your brain a chance to hit the "refresh" button on a bad memory. Typically with a trained therapist, you begin moving your eyes from side to side or tapping your knees in a rhythmic way to activate both sides of your brain while thinking about a traumatic event. It's like reprogramming your brain to handle that memory differently so it's no longer stuck on repeat in your head. It's structured, yes, but super effective for helping your brain process trauma in a new way. Keep in mind that if you have done EMDR with a practitioner for a while and feel comfortable doing so, you can give this a try on your own. I have added some online platforms to the resource page.

### *The Butterfly Hug EMDR Exercise*

Here's a simplified version of an EMDR exercise that can help you work through a distressing memory. While this isn't a substitute for working with a trained EMDR therapist, it offers a glimpse of how you might use bilateral stimulation to process emotions.

**Purpose:** This exercise uses bilateral stimulation (activating both sides of your brain) to help reduce the emotional intensity of a distressing memory or thought. It combines the basic principle of EMDR—processing trauma by engaging both sides of the brain—with self-soothing through a gentle, calming practice.

### *Instructions:*

1. **Make sure you are resting comfortably:** Sit and be in a safe place where you won't be disturbed. Take three deep cleansing breaths to balance yourself and bring your awareness to the present. Allow yourself to feel grounded and supported in your space.

2. **Identify a distressing memory or thought:** Think of a recent memory or thought that has caused you distress. Choose something that feels manageable to

work with—something that stirs up some discomfort but not so overwhelming that it feels unbearable.

3. **Rate your distress:** On a scale of 0 to 10, where 0 is no distress, and 10 is the highest level of distress, rate how upset you feel when you think about this memory or thought. This will help you track your progress as you move through the exercise.

4. **The butterfly hug:** Cross your arms over your chest so that your fingertips are resting on the opposite shoulders—this forms the "butterfly wings." Once you're in this position, begin tapping your hands alternately on your shoulders, left-right-left-right. Do this at a comfortable pace, about three taps per second. This is your bilateral stimulation.

5. **Focus on the memory and tap:** As you tap, bring your attention to the distressing memory or thought. Allow yourself to notice any emotions, body sensations, or images that come up as you think about it. Keep tapping and breathing steadily as you observe what comes up. There's no need to force anything—just let your mind and body process whatever comes naturally. It is normal to experience random thoughts like, "What should I have for dinner?" Notice them, but keep tapping.

6. **Notice shifts:** Continue tapping and focusing on the memory for one minute. Afterward, pause and check in with yourself. Notice if anything has shifted—whether your emotions, body sensations, or thoughts have changed in any way. You may feel a reduction in distress or notice new thoughts or feelings emerging.

7. **Rate your distress again:** After a round of tapping, rate your distress level again on the 0-10 scale. Has it

decreased? If you still feel a significant level of distress, repeat the tapping process, focusing on the memory and allowing your mind and body to process it.

8. **Replace the memory with a positive thought:** Once your distress has reduced to a manageable level, shift your focus to a positive thought or an image that plasters a smile across your face. It could be something that brings you peace, joy, or a sense of strength. Begin tapping again, this time focusing on this positive thought or image. Let the bilateral stimulation reinforce this new, positive association.

9. **Reflect and rest:** When you're ready, stop tapping and take a few moments to rest. Take a few deep breaths and gently bring your awareness back to the present moment. Reflect on the exercise and any shifts that occurred. Ask yourself:

    o How do you feel now compared to when you started?

_____
_____
_____
_____
_____

## *Why This Helps*

This exercise mimics the bilateral stimulation used in EMDR therapy, helping your brain process distressing memories or thoughts in a more balanced way—like a yoga session for your psyche! By engaging both sides of your brain through the Butterfly Hug, you can reduce the intensity of negative emotions and replace them with more positive associations, creating a mental garden where sunny thoughts can blossom.

You can whip this exercise out whenever you feel the need to process a difficult memory or emotion. It's a simple yet powerful tool to help you soothe yourself and glide through distress in a safe and supportive way, like a warm hug for your mind!

## *Polyvagal Theory*

Polyvagal Theory, developed by Dr. Stephen Porges, is a groundbreaking approach that helps us understand how our nervous system responds to stress, trauma, and social connection. It's all about how our autonomic nervous system—the part of us that works behind the scenes, keeping us alive—controls our reactions to the world around us.

The theory focuses on three primary states of the nervous system (*Polyvagal Therapy*, 2018):

1. **Social Engagement (Ventral Vagal State):** This is our "safe and snuggly" state. When we're here, we feel like we just won the social lottery—calm, connected, and ready for some heartfelt banter. Think of the cozy vibes when you're curled up with a loved one or indulge in your favorite guilty pleasure.

2. **Fight or Flight (Sympathetic State):** Welcome to our "ready, set, panic!" mode. This kicks in when we sense danger, making us choose between booking it out of there or standing our ground. It's our body's built-in alarm system, but if we get trapped here, anxiety, panic, and chronic stress become our unwanted party guests.

3. **Shutdown (Dorsal Vagal State):** Ah, the "freeze or fizzle" state. When threats start feeling like an avalanche, our system hits the brakes and goes into

shutdown. It can leave us feeling numb, disconnected, and ready to audition for a role in a drama about despair. It's our defense mechanism when the notion of fight-or-flight seems more like a bad sitcom.

Polyvagal Theory is used in somatic therapy to help people become more aware of which state their nervous system is in and to guide them back to a place of safety and connection. The goal is to help the nervous system become more flexible and adaptable so that you can navigate stress and trauma more effectively.

## *Polyvagal Exercise: The Safe and Sound Anchor*

This exercise helps you activate your ventral vagal state (your "safe and connected" state) by creating a sense of safety in your body. It's all about grounding yourself in the present moment and shifting your nervous system back into a state where you can engage with the world from a place of calm.

**Purpose:** The goal of this exercise is to help you feel more grounded and connected by activating your ventral vagal state, which promotes relaxation, social engagement, and a sense of safety. It's a simple way to soothe your nervous system when you're feeling anxious or disconnected.

## *Instructions:*

1. **Get cozy:** Make sure you are comfortable and you feel safe. This could be your favorite chair, a cozy spot on the couch, or anywhere that feels like a "safe zone" for you. Take a moment to notice your surroundings and let yourself settle into the present moment.

2. **Engage with your breath:** Start by paying attention to your breath. You don't need to change it; just notice

it. Feel the air coming in and going out. If you're comfortable, place one hand on your heart and the other on your belly. This helps create a feeling of connection with yourself.

3. **Activate your senses:** Begin to engage your senses one by one. Notice what you can see around you—colors, shapes, light. Then, listen to the sounds in your environment, both close and far away. Next, focus on what you can feel—the texture of your clothes, the ground beneath you, or the warmth of your hands on your body. Take a moment to notice any scents or tastes in the air. This gentle engagement with your senses can help anchor you in the present moment.

4. **Create a safe and sound anchor:** Think of something that makes you feel safe and connected. It could be a memory of being with a loved one, a favorite place, or even a comforting image. Hold that thought or image in your mind, and notice how your body responds. Do you feel warmth in your chest? A softening of your muscles? Stay with this feeling for a few moments, allowing it to expand and fill your body.

5. **Vocalization or humming:** Humming is a simple way to activate your ventral vagal nerve and bring yourself into a state of calm. Try humming softly, noticing the gentle vibration in your chest and throat. This vibration helps to soothe your nervous system. If you prefer, you can also try singing a few lines of a favorite song or even repeating a calming phrase or word out loud. The sound of your own voice can help you feel more connected to yourself and others.

6. **Notice the shift:** After spending some time with this exercise, take a moment to notice any shifts in your body and emotions. Do you feel more relaxed or

connected? Has your breathing slowed down? If you feel safe and calm, stay with this feeling as long as you like. If not, it's okay to repeat the exercise or move at your own pace.

7. **Reflection:** When you're ready, gently bring your awareness back to your surroundings. Reflect on how you feel now compared to when you started. Is there a difference in your level of calmness or connection? Carry this sense of safety with you as you move forward with your day.

*Why This Helps*

This exercise engages your ventral vagal state, helping to bring you out of fight-or-flight or shutdown mode and into a state of safety and social engagement. By focusing on your breath, senses, and a safe image, you help your nervous system feel more connected and calm. This can be a helpful tool whenever you're feeling anxious, overwhelmed, or disconnected.

Each of these therapies focuses on the body, but they approach healing in different ways. Whether you need to shake off trauma like a deer, feel your emotions with a trusted guide, rewrite old body patterns, rewire your brain, or just learn to be more present, there's a somatic therapy out there that can help. It's like finding the right tool in the toolbox for your specific healing journey.

# The Benefits of Somatic Practices

Now, let's talk about the benefits of engaging in regular movement. You may have heard the phrase "move it or lose it," and it holds true in this context: Regular movement prevents energy stagnation. Imagine your body as a river. A flowing river is clear and life-giving, providing nourishment and habitat to countless organisms. In contrast, a stagnant body of water becomes murky and supports little life. Have you ever seen a river clogged up with debris like fallen trees and such? Immediately, that beautiful flow of water has issues and becomes backed up, right?

Similarly, when you keep your body in motion, you prevent the buildup of stagnant energy that could lead to emotional muddiness and physical discomfort. Regular physical activity keeps the energy channels open, making sure that stagnant emotions don't get a chance to settle in. Your river won't get clogged up with debris.

Engaging in consistent movement practices isn't just a way to maintain physical fitness but also a means to promote emotional health. Exercise releases endorphins—the body's natural mood lifters. These chemicals help you feel happier and more at ease, which means you're not only working out physical stress but also improving your mental state. Think of moments when you've felt particularly low or anxious, and recall how even a short walk had the power to lift your spirits. That's the emotional benefit of keeping your body moving consistently.

Incorporating movement into your daily routine doesn't mean you have to commit to hours at the gym or rigorous workouts. Simple activities like walking, stretching, or even dancing around your living room can be immensely beneficial. The key here is consistency rather than intensity. Find what works best for you and stick with it. Over time, you'll notice not only physical improvements but also a heightened sense of emotional well-being.

## The Effectiveness of Somatic Practices

The effectiveness of somatic practices is increasingly supported by scientific evidence, highlighting their significant benefits for mental and physical health. One of the key areas where somatic practices have shown promise is in reducing symptoms of PTSD and anxiety. Research has found that engaging in activities such as yoga, mindfulness meditation, and body-oriented therapies can help alleviate the distressing symptoms associated with these conditions (Kuhfuß et al., 2021).

For instance, a study involving veterans suffering from PTSD demonstrated that a structured yoga program helped reduce both the severity and frequency of their symptoms. Participants reported decreased hyperarousal and intrusive thoughts, and an overall improvement in mood and sleep quality (Chopin et al., 2020). These findings suggest that incorporating somatic practices into your routine could be beneficial if you are coping with similar issues.

Physical activities like exercise and yoga are not only beneficial for mental health but also strengthen resilience. Regular physical activity has long been known to release endorphins, which are chemicals in your brain that act as natural painkillers and mood elevators. Studies have shown that regular involvement in aerobic exercises, including running, swimming, and cycling, can greatly improve mental health outcomes (Sharma et al., 2006). Yoga, with its combination of physical poses, breathing techniques, and meditation, offers a holistic approach that strengthens both mind and body.

For example, research indicates that people who engage in regular physical activity have lower rates of depression and anxiety than those who do not (Sharma et al., 2006). This suggests that even simple actions like taking a daily walk or joining a local exercise class are important in maintaining mental health resilience. If you incorporate such activities into your routine, you might notice an improved ability to cope with stress and a heightened sense of well-being.

Somatic therapies also contribute to long-term improvements in emotional regulation and stress management. Therapies such as Somatic Experiencing and Sensorimotor Psychotherapy are specifically designed to address the trauma stored in your body. These approaches often involve mindful awareness of bodily sensations and fostering a sense of safety within your body, which can help you process and release pent-up emotions (Jones, 2022).

Scientific studies support the use of these therapies for improving emotional regulation. For instance, patients undergoing Somatic Experiencing reported significant reductions in PTSD symptoms and better emotional control over time (Almeida et al., 2020). By learning to connect with your body and understand its signals, you can develop healthier ways to handle stress and regulate your mood.

Positive physiological changes are another critical benefit observed in those practicing somatic techniques regularly. One notable change is the reduction of cortisol levels. Cortisol, often referred to as the "stress hormone," plays a crucial role in your body's response to stress. Elevated cortisol levels, however, can lead to various adverse health effects, including weight gain, high blood pressure, and impaired cognitive function.

Research has shown that somatic practices, such as yoga, tai chi, and Qigong, can significantly lower cortisol levels (Rogerson et al., 2023). Regular practice of such techniques can help maintain a lower cortisol baseline, improving overall health. Integrating these practices into your life, you may experience less stress and a more balanced physiological state.

Other physiological benefits include improvements in heart rate variability (HRV), which is an indicator of autonomic nervous system functioning. Higher HRV is associated with greater resilience to stress and better cardiovascular health. Practicing deep breathing exercises, meditation, and gentle physical movements, common in many somatic practices, has been shown to enhance HRV, further supporting mental and physical well-being.

# Integrating Somatic Practices Into Daily Routines

Consistency is key for reaping the benefits of somatic practices. Consider these tips for making them a regular part of your life:

- **Set a schedule:** Dedicate specific times of the day for your practices. Morning routines can energize you for the day ahead, while evening sessions can promote relaxation and better sleep.

- **Be flexible:** Allow for flexibility in your routine. If you miss a session, don't stress—just pick up where you left off next time.

- **Combine practices:** Mix and match different somatic practices. For instance, you might start your day with a butterfly hug exercise and wind down in the evening with polyvagal vagus nerve stimulation.

## *Post-Activity Care*

After engaging in any somatic practice, it's important to take care of your body to maximize benefits and prevent any adverse effects. Here are some tips:

- **Hydration:** Drink plenty of water before and after your practice to stay hydrated. Water helps flush out toxins released during physical activity.

- **Rest:** Give yourself time to rest and recover. This could be through a short nap or simply sitting quietly and letting your body unwind.

- **Reflection:** Spend a few minutes reflecting on your experience. Journaling can be a helpful way to process your emotions and track your progress.

# Final Thoughts

Remember, the goal of somatic healing is to create space for your body to express and release what it has been holding onto. Whether it's through co-regulation with a loved one or receiving a massage, each method emphasizes the importance of tuning into your body's signals. When you consistently practice these techniques, you'll be empowering yourself to heal from within and cultivate a deeper sense of emotional, mental, and physical peace. So take the time to explore and honor what your body needs—your healing path is uniquely yours.

It's time to move on to the next chapter of "Oops, I've Packed My Trauma," where we will explore what breathwork is, the importance of diaphragmatic breathing, and how you can use them both to heal your trauma and calm your nervous system.

# Chapter 7:
# Polarity Therapy

Ever felt like your body's energy is more scrambled than a chaotic morning commute? You're not alone. When life gets busy, it's easy for your energy to go haywire, leaving you feeling drained, off-balance, and stuck in a funk. That's where polarity therapy steps in, like a Zen traffic cop, gently guiding your energy back into harmony.

It is time to walk through the four foundations of polarity therapy and show you how each one plays a role in calming your energy. No fluff, no jargon—just practical, relatable examples of how this modality can help you feel more balanced, healthy, and in control of your energy.

## An Introduction to Polarity Therapy

Developed by Dr. Randolph Stone, an American osteopathic physician with a keen interest in ancient wisdom, polarity therapy is all about getting that energy flowing smoothly again (*Who Developed Polarity Therapy?*, 2014).

Dr. Stone, who blended his love for spiritual and mystic texts from Indian and Hebrew traditions with his medical expertise, wanted to figure out what really caused pain and disease. He discovered that energy flow—known as "prana" in Ayurveda, an ancient Indian medical system—was the key. So, he created polarity therapy to bridge these ancient Eastern concepts and the

Western mindset. It's like blending yoga with a modern dance party!

In the 1940s, Dr. Stone introduced polarity therapy to his clients in Chicago after spending decades researching energy healing techniques worldwide. His approach incorporated practices like Ayurveda, Chinese medicine, reflexology, and even Hermetic philosophy. He wasn't just thinking "body"—he saw the connection between the physical, emotional, mental, and energetic aspects of well-being (*Who Developed Polarity Therapy?*, 2014). It's a whole-body experience, not just a quick fix for an achy shoulder.

Now, let's clear up a common question: Is polarity therapy like massage therapy or Reiki? Not exactly! Massage focuses on working your muscles and loosening up tension, while Reiki is about channeling universal energy into the body through a practitioner's hands. Polarity therapy, on the other hand, is like the gentle conductor of your body's energy symphony. It uses non-invasive touch and awareness to encourage the natural flow of energy in your body. Instead of focusing on just the muscles or channeling energy, it tunes in to the big picture—your energy as a whole—and helps restore balance.

So, if you've ever felt out of sync, like your energy is stuck in a traffic jam, polarity therapy might just be the thing to get your body's dance party back on track.

## The Main Goal of Polarity Therapy

Polarity therapy's main goal is to restore balance and harmony to your body's energy flow. When your energy pathways get blocked or out of sync, you may experience physical pain, emotional stress, or even illness. Polarity therapy has the goal of getting everything moving again!

Polarity therapy can be used for a wide variety of issues—physical, emotional, and mental. From chronic pain, stress, and digestive problems to emotional challenges like anxiety and trauma, polarity therapy is like a jack-of-all-trades. It's particularly useful for those times when you feel like everything is just... off.

Through a combination of bodywork, counseling, nutritional guidance, and exercise, polarity therapy helps to clear out those energy blockages and restore flow. Think of it as a multi-tool for your health.

## How Does a Practitioner Become Certified?

Becoming a certified polarity therapist is no walk in the park. It requires 800 hours of training—yep, that's more than enough time to binge-watch every season of your favorite show (twice). After the training, they must pass an exam to become a Board Certified Polarity Practitioner (BCPP) issued by the American Polarity Therapy Association (Pistoia, 2022).

## The Four Principles of Polarity Therapy

Polarity therapy stands on four main pillars: counseling, bodywork, nutrition, and exercise. These principles work together like a superhero squad to keep your body's energy balanced and harmonious.

## Counseling: The Mind-Energy Connection

Counseling in polarity therapy isn't the same as traditional talk therapy. Instead, it's about exploring how your thoughts and emotions affect your energy flow. Picture your mind as the control room for your body's energy. When it's filled with negative thoughts, it's like sending out bad vibes that block your energy flow. Counseling helps you recognize and shift these thoughts to keep your energy highways clear.

Your therapist will use active and reflective listening to help you become more aware of the patterns in your life that might be creating those blockages. It's not about deep psychological work but rather about making you more mindful of the connection between your mind and energy.

## Bodywork: Freeing the Flow

Bodywork is the bread and butter of polarity therapy. Imagine your body as a garden hose—sometimes, life's stresses create those pesky kinks that stop the water (or, in this case, energy) from flowing freely. Bodywork is like the gentle hands that untangle those knots, allowing your energy to move smoothly throughout your body again.

During a session, your therapist might use light touch, gentle rocking, or even stretches to help release these energy blockages. It's a bit like hitting a reset button for your body's energy system. You'll often walk away from a session feeling lighter, more relaxed, and with a sense of fluidity in your movements and emotions. It's about restoring balance, so your energy flows as it should—effortlessly and naturally.

## *Nutrition: Feeding Your Energy*

In polarity therapy, nutrition isn't just about what you put on your plate; it's about how the food you eat influences the flow of energy within your body. Forget calorie counting or restrictive diets—this is about nourishing your energy with the kind of food that fuels your entire being.

Think of whole foods like fruits, vegetables, and anti-inflammatory spices as the premium fuel your body craves. When you steer clear of toxins—like artificial additives and processed junk—you're essentially clearing the path for your energy to flow freely. Nutrition in polarity therapy is all about feeding your body the clean, vibrant fuel it needs to thrive, helping you feel more energized, balanced, and in tune with yourself.

## *Exercise: Moving Your Energy*

Exercise in polarity therapy isn't about hitting the gym or running marathons. It's more about gentle, instinctual movements that help keep your energy in motion. Imagine doing yoga-like stretches that feel natural to your body, with a bit of vocal expression thrown in—like saying "ha" or "hum" while stretching out tension.

These simple movements are like energy tunes, keeping your body's flow in harmony. Even just a few minutes a day can make a difference, helping you feel more balanced and energized.

Polarity therapy is unique to everyone. It is a personalized roadmap to restore peace and calm in your body and mind. Through counseling, bodywork, nutrition, and exercise, you can clear those energy blockages and get back to feeling like your best self. And the best part? It's all about reconnecting with yourself in a way that feels natural, light-hearted, and maybe even a little fun.

# A Polarity Session Up Close

Picture this: You're sitting in a cozy room with soft lighting and peaceful music in the background. You're here for your first polarity therapy session, unsure of what to expect but hopeful that it might help you feel more like... well, you again. That's exactly where Charles found himself not too long ago.

Charles, a middle-aged man juggling work stress and family responsibilities, found himself drowning in anxiety. His trauma stemmed from a major boating accident that happened two years ago. Ever since then, he'd been struggling with trouble sleeping, constant tension in his shoulders, and an inability to focus at work. No matter what he tried—therapy, meditation apps, even long jogs—nothing seemed to break through the fog. He felt stuck in a loop of worry and exhaustion.

Enter polarity therapy.

## *The Interview: Discussing Charles' Needs*

When Charles first met with his polarity therapist, the session didn't start with bodywork. Instead, they had a heart-to-heart. His therapist asked him to describe his current experience—what brought him here? What was he hoping to achieve? Charles talked about his sleepless nights, his constant state of tension, and his wish to stop feeling like a hamster on a never-ending wheel.

The therapist listened closely, nodding and taking notes. This was the time for Charles to feel seen and heard, which, let's be real, is already a form of therapy in itself.

## *Assessing Charles' Energy State*

Next, the therapist began assessing Charles' energy state. Remember, polarity therapy is all about the flow of energy in your body. Charles' therapist used gentle touch and observation to sense where his energy might be stuck. His upper body felt heavy, especially around his chest and shoulders—classic signs of stored stress and anxiety. His lower body, in contrast, felt like it needed grounding.

Charles felt a little skeptical at first. Energy? He wasn't sure how to measure that. But he trusted the process.

## *Applying Polarity Therapy Techniques*

Then came the actual bodywork. Charles remained fully clothed, lying on a massage table, and his therapist began using light touch, rocking movements, and pressure on specific points of his body. It wasn't like a deep-tissue massage but more like a gentle nudge to his energy system.

At one point, Charles felt warmth in his hands and, at another, a tingling in his feet. The therapist explained that this was his energy responding, shifting to where it needed to go. Charles might not have fully understood it, but he did feel an odd sense of relaxation wash over him—something he hadn't felt in months.

Throughout the session, the therapist checked in with Charles, asking how he felt, adjusting pressure where needed, and encouraging him to breathe deeply. It wasn't a one-size-fits-all experience. If something felt too intense or uncomfortable, they backed off. The whole idea was to meet Charles where he was, energetically and emotionally.

## *The First Month: Charles' Journey*

Charles committed to trying polarity therapy for a month, which meant weekly sessions. After his first session, he slept better than he had in weeks. He wasn't "cured" overnight, but he noticed small shifts. He felt a little less tense at work, and his thoughts didn't race as much. By his third session, Charles found himself looking forward to his appointments. He used some of the breathing techniques his therapist recommended in his daily life, especially during stressful meetings.

Were there cons? Well, Charles found it a little difficult at first to explain to friends what polarity therapy was all about. Some raised an eyebrow when he mentioned "energy work." And, like anything, he had to remind himself to stay consistent. There were days when he felt too busy for a session, but those were often the days he needed it the most.

By the end of the month, Charles wasn't just sleeping better; he felt more in control. His anxiety didn't vanish, but it stopped ruling his life. He felt more grounded, more balanced—like his energy was flowing in the right direction again.

What did Charles take away from his month of sessions? The biggest lesson was that energy isn't some mysterious force beyond his control—it's something he could work with. He used simple techniques, like grounding exercises and breathwork, to manage his anxiety when it flared up. It wasn't always easy, but knowing he had tools at his disposal made all the difference.

Charles' time with polarity therapy showed him that healing isn't just about fixing symptoms; it's about creating balance. It's about working with your body, your energy, and emotions in a way that feels gentle and supportive. And yes, sometimes that means stepping into the unknown and trusting the process.

## Polarity Therapy at Home

Let's walk through how Chelsea uses polarity therapy at home.

Chelsea sat on her yoga mat in the middle of her living room, taking a deep breath. It had been six months since the pregnancy loss, and the weight of it still pressed down on her chest. Every day, she tried to push through, but her body and mind were drained and exhausted. The stress, the grief, it all seemed to settle deep in her muscles, like she couldn't release it, no matter how many times she tried.

Her naturopath had suggested polarity therapy, and while Chelsea had seen a practitioner, she needed something she could do at home when those heavy moments crept in. That's when she remembered the exercises her practitioner recommended—

simple but powerful moves that could help balance her body's energy.

*"Okay, Chelsea,"* she whispered to herself. *"Let's do this."*

## *Keeping Your Body Balanced: The Squat*

Chelsea stood up, grounding herself with her feet shoulder-width apart. She started with the squat. It seemed simple enough, but this wasn't just about working out—this was about reconnecting with her body.

1. Stand tall with your feet shoulder-width apart, turning them slightly outward. She exhaled, trying to let go of some tension.

2. Slowly, Chelsea squatted down as far as she could, making sure her knees stayed in line with her feet. It wasn't easy at first—her muscles were tight, her body resistant as if it didn't want to let go of the grief. But she allowed herself to sink into the pose, letting the stretch deepen naturally.

3. The hard part? Staying there and holding for a full minute. Chelsea felt the burn in her thighs, but as the seconds ticked by, she also felt something shift—like her body was beginning to release some of that stored tension. Not all of it, but enough to breathe a little easier.

When she finally stood back up, she shook out her legs and smiled. *That wasn't so bad,* she thought. For a moment, she felt grounded, as if the simple act of squatting had somehow helped her stand taller, too.

## Ridding Yourself of Stress: The Woodchopper

Next, it was time for the woodchopper. The name made Chelsea chuckle. *Maybe I should imagine chopping all this stress away,* she mused.

1. Feet slightly wider than shoulder-width apart. Inhale, Chelsea raised her arms overhead like she was holding an imaginary axe. She could almost hear her husband's voice in the back of her mind: "Be careful with that thing!" She smiled.

2. On the exhale, she brought her hands down quickly between her legs, imagining the chop. The motion felt cathartic—like she was cutting through the weight she'd been carrying. She did it again, breathing in, raising her hands, then chopping down as she exhaled, faster this time. By the tenth repetition, her breath was coming faster, but so was her heartbeat—energized, lighter.

## Proper Nutrition and Staying Balanced

As Chelsea cooled down, she remembered another thing her practitioner had mentioned: nutrition. It wasn't just about exercises—balance needed to happen from the inside out. Lately, she'd been surviving on coffee and quick snacks, but maybe it was time to nourish herself differently.

"Okay, body," she said out loud. "Time for a reset. More water, more veggies, fewer late-night cookie binges." She laughed because she knew that last one would be tough. She took the time to make herself a healthy snack of raw vegetables and hummus. She drank some water and reflected on her session.

Today, after these simple exercises, Chelsea felt something she hadn't in a while—hope. It wasn't a cure-all, and it wouldn't bring her baby back, but it was a start. A small step toward healing, one squat, one woodchop, and one healthy snack at a time.

And so, she continued day by day, finding little ways to balance herself at home, discovering that even in the darkest times, the light could find a way back in if she let it.

# Is Polarity Effective?

You may be wondering if this is all just a bunch of nice stories or if there's any actual science behind it. That's where the research comes in. In a small 2019 study, researchers examined the effect of four polarity therapy sessions on middle-aged women who struggled with anxiety and insomnia. The results? The women who received the treatment saw an evident improvement compared to those who didn't. It was like a breath of fresh air for these women, allowing them to sleep more peacefully and feel calmer in their daily lives (Lambert et al., 2019).

There was a study done in 2011 that looked at the impact of polarity therapy on cancer-related fatigue in 45 women undergoing radiation therapy for breast cancer. Polarity therapy helped reduce the extreme exhaustion these women felt, showing that energy work can be a powerful ally even during such a challenging time (Mustian et al., 2011).

But it doesn't stop there. In 2012, researchers wanted to see if polarity therapy could help reduce stress in caregivers looking after people with dementia—because let's face it, caregiving is emotionally and physically draining. They had 42 participants who either underwent eight sessions of polarity therapy or participated in other relaxing activities like yoga or even basket weaving.

The results were telling. Those who underwent polarity therapy had big reductions in stress levels and depression compared to the other participants (Korn et al., 2012).

# Final Thoughts

Ultimately, polarity therapy offers you a way to reconnect with your body and energy in a deeply healing way. It's about helping your body do what it's naturally designed to do: heal, release, and find balance. Whether you're dealing with stress, physical pain, or emotional trauma, polarity therapy gives you a chance to lighten that load and start feeling like yourself again.

What is up next? The art of breathwork! Let's take a closer look at the powerful tool of breathwork and how it can release stored trauma.

# Chapter 8:
# Finding Stillness Through Breathwork

Have you ever found yourself holding your breath during a stressful or anxious moment, only to realize that you've been stuck in that tense state for hours, days, maybe even years? Yeah, me too. It's wild how we can carry tension around like an old suitcase, crammed full of stuff we don't even need anymore. Breathwork can help us unpack that suitcase, one calming breath at a time.

The goal of this chapter is to explore how to use breathwork as a tool to release stored trauma and restore balance. Maybe you're feeling overwhelmed by emotions or just trying to calm your busy mind. I'll walk you through some simple exercises, share a few stories from people just like you, and throw in some light-hearted tips to help you find that stillness within. You're going to feel a lot lighter by the end of this. Are you ready to breathe easier?

## Breathwork Fundamentals: Breathe In, Breathe Out, Heal

Let's start with something simple. You're doing it right now without even thinking—breathing. The thing is, when you start paying attention to your breath, it becomes a powerful tool for healing. Breathwork is like that one app on your phone that you didn't know could change your life, but it's been there all along, just waiting for you to click it.

Breathwork is the conscious control of your breath to influence your mental, emotional, and physical state. Think of it as a remote control for your inner world, and you get to decide if it's time for a rerun of calm and relaxation or a brand-new episode of deep healing. Whether it's a long, slow inhale or a quick, energizing exhale, different breathwork techniques can produce different effects.

These methods aren't new—people have been using breathwork for centuries in spiritual practices like yoga, meditation, and qi gong. Ancient cultures knew what they were doing when it came to tapping into the power of breath.

Yogic breathing, or pranayama, has been a cornerstone of Indian traditions for centuries. If you've ever taken a yoga class and found yourself huffing and puffing during the breathing exercises, congratulations—you've dipped your toes into pranayama. Then there's holotropic breathwork, developed in the 1970s by psychiatrist Stanislav Grof, which uses accelerated breathing to reach altered states of consciousness (Russell, 2021). This one's like taking a deep dive into the ocean of your subconscious, fishing for insights and emotional release.

Now, let's get into why this matters for trauma recovery. When we experience trauma, our body's natural response is often to hold on to the stress—tight muscles, shallow breathing, a general sense of being on edge. Breathwork helps you do the opposite. It invites you to release that pent-up tension and shift out of fight-or-flight mode. Think of it like this: You're opening a pressure valve that's been stuck for far too long.

Take Jason, for example. Jason had been carrying trauma from his childhood—neglect and abandonment issues—that lingered, no matter how much he tried to ignore them. He turned to breathwork as a last-ditch effort. Through regular sessions of conscious connected breathing, Josh noticed something amazing—his body finally started to let go. He felt lighter, less burdened by his past. And this wasn't just in his head. He could feel the difference physically. His shoulders dropped, his jaw unclenched, and for the first time in a long time, he could breathe deeply without feeling like a weight was sitting on his chest.

So, if you're wondering how breathwork could help you, imagine using your breath as a tool to clear out the cobwebs of your trauma. It's about giving yourself permission to let go, release, and finally take in a deep, healing breath of fresh air.

In a world where we're always holding on to something—stress, emotions, even physical tension—breathwork is your invitation to let go. It's not just about oxygenating your body (though that's a nice bonus); it's about giving yourself the space to heal from the inside out. Breath by breath.

## The Role of Breath in Healing

Breath is one of those things we do without thinking—until we realize that it's so much more than just filling our lungs with air. Breath is inherently connected to our emotional state, whether we're aware of it or not. Think about how you breathe when you're stressed or anxious—short, shallow, and rapid. Now, contrast that with how you breathe when you're relaxed—slow, deep, and rhythmic. This connection between breath and emotions is why breath is such a powerful tool for healing trauma.

When you consciously use your breath, you can foster a sense of safety and promote emotional release. It's like having a built-in reset button. Imagine you've had a tough day, and your mind is swirling with all the stress and overwhelm. But then you sit down, close your eyes, and take a deep, slow breath in. You hold it for a moment and then let it out slowly. With each exhale, it's like you're releasing a little bit of that tension, like letting the air out of a balloon that's been blown up too tight. This simple act of focusing on your breath can make you feel more grounded, more in control, and safer in your own body.

Breath awareness builds mindfulness, which is important for trauma recovery. Here's an example: Let's say you've experienced something really tough in your life, and that experience left you feeling disconnected from yourself. You might find it hard to be present in the moment because your mind keeps pulling you back to the past. But when you bring your attention to your breath, you pull yourself into the present. You remind yourself that you are here, right now, and that the past no longer has control over you. You can start small, like noticing how the air feels as it enters your nostrils and fills your lungs. Little by little, this awareness of breath brings you back to yourself, helping you reclaim your power over your own body and emotions.

## *Basic Mechanics of Breathing*

Alright, let's break down how breathing actually works—because, believe it or not, there's more to it than just "in and out." When you breathe, your diaphragm (a dome-shaped muscle under your lungs) contracts and moves downward, allowing your lungs to expand and fill with air. This is your body's way of bringing in oxygen, which is crucial for pretty much everything that happens inside you, from thinking to digesting to, yes, healing. On the exhale, your diaphragm relaxes, and air is pushed out of your lungs, releasing carbon dioxide (Vorvick, 2023). This cycle of inhalation and exhalation is your body's way of maintaining balance. But here's where it gets interesting: Your breathing patterns are closely tied to your emotional state. Ever notice how your breath gets shallow when you're anxious or scared?

That's because your body is preparing for a fight-or-flight response. It's like your breath is saying, "We've got to stay alert!" But the thing is, when your breath stays in that shallow, rapid state for too long, it can keep you stuck in that heightened state of stress, which isn't doing your body or your healing any favors.

When you understand the mechanics of breathing, you can start to work with your breath more effectively. For example, knowing that deep, diaphragmatic breathing (that's the belly-breathing kind) activates your parasympathetic nervous system—the part that helps you relax—you can use this knowledge to shift yourself out of stress mode and into a more relaxed state. Think of it as a little hack for calming your body and mind, all through the simple act of breathing.

## *Importance of Intentional Breathing*

When it comes to intentional breathing, it's like giving your body a gentle reminder: "Hey, we're on the same team!" Imagine yourself sitting down after a stressful day, feeling the tension in your shoulders and that pit in your stomach. Now, think about what happens when you just stop and take a deep breath—not just any breath, but one with purpose. That's what intentional breathing is all about. You're not just sucking in air; you're directing your breath to create a shift in how you feel, both mentally and physically.

Intentional breathing is like a bridge between your mind and body, helping you tap into that hidden superpower called healing. When you breathe with intention, you're sending a message to your body: "It's okay to let go." And your body listens! Your heart rate slows down, your muscles relax, and suddenly, that stress monster doesn't seem so big anymore. It's like your breath becomes this magical key that unlocks the door to healing.

But it's more than just calming down. Intentional breathing allows you to set a personal intention, which makes the whole experience more powerful. For example, let's say you're struggling with feelings of self-worth. By breathing intentionally, focusing on self-love with each inhale, and releasing doubt with each exhale, you're creating a mini ritual that strengthens your emotional healing. It's rooted in the way our brains and bodies work together.

So, how do you align your breath with your emotional healing goals? Start by asking yourself: "What do I need right now?" If you're feeling overwhelmed, your intention could be to find calm. If you're struggling with past trauma, your intention might be to let go. With each breath, focus on that goal.

Maybe your goal is to release anger or to invite more joy into your life. With every inhale, visualize yourself drawing in what you need. With every exhale, imagine letting go of what's holding you back. Start small, like setting aside just a few minutes each day to breathe intentionally, aligning your breath with what you want to heal.

When you focus on your breath with purpose, you're not just breathing—you're actively participating in your healing. And trust me, it feels amazing to realize that something as simple as breathing can be so transformative.

# The Benefits and Science Behind Breathwork

You might think breathwork sounds like something only practiced by deep-sea divers or monks sitting on mountaintops, but it's actually something incredibly accessible to you right now. And trust me, your body and mind will thank you for it. Here's why.

### *Physiological Benefits: Relax Your Body, Revive Your Life*

Have you ever been stuck in traffic, hands gripping the steering wheel, and you're late for an important meeting? Your breath is shallow, your heart's pounding, and stress hormones are firing on all cylinders. Now imagine that same scenario, but instead, you take a slow, deep breath in through your nose, hold it for a moment, and gently exhale through your mouth. Ahh, suddenly, that tension releases, and you feel more in control. That's the art of breathwork.

Breathwork isn't just about feeling Zen; it has real, physiological effects on your body. Studies show that deep breathing activates your parasympathetic nervous system—the part of your body that tells you to "chill out." When you take those slow, deliberate breaths, it lowers cortisol (your stress hormone), reducing anxiety and promoting relaxation. One study even found that participants who practiced breathwork experienced a significant reduction in their cortisol levels by nearly 20% (Zaccaro et al., 2018). That's like turning down the volume on your stress.

But it's not just about calming your nerves. Breathwork also increases oxygen flow, which can boost your physical vitality and mental clarity. Think of it like filling up your body's gas tank—more oxygen means more energy to tackle whatever life throws your way. And when your brain gets more oxygen? Hello, clearer thinking and focus! In fact, studies show that simple deep breathing exercises can increase brain activity in the prefrontal cortex, the area responsible for decision-making and focus (Zaccaro et al., 2018). So, next time you're about to have a challenging conversation or need a boost of energy, remember to take that deep breath.

## *Psychological Benefits: Healing From the Inside Out*

Let's get real—trauma and stress aren't just in your head; they're stored in your body, too. Your breath is a bridge between your body and mind, and tapping into it can unlock some serious emotional release. When you engage in breathwork, you're giving your body the tools to heal from within, managing symptoms of anxiety, depression, and even PTSD. It's like giving your emotional baggage a one-way ticket out of your body!

Imagine being able to regulate those overwhelming emotions with just a few minutes of focused breathing. Research shows that breathwork can enhance your emotional resilience, giving you the strength to face difficult situations without feeling completely overwhelmed (Montes & Penzenstadler, 2023). One study highlighted that people who practiced breathwork reported fewer symptoms of anxiety and depression after just a few weeks (Banushi et al., 2023). So, if you've ever felt like your emotions are a runaway train, breathwork might just be the brake you need.

Studies have shown that breathwork can alter brain activity, specifically increasing alpha waves, which are associated with relaxation and emotional release (Banushi et al., 2023). Essentially, when you breathe deeply, you're not just calming your mind; you're literally changing your brain chemistry. This makes it easier to let go of pent-up emotions and stress.

One fascinating study published in the *Frontiers in Psychology* journal found that participants who engaged in controlled breathwork experienced huge improvements in emotional regulation and cognitive function (Zaccaro et al., 2018). That's because breathwork helps balance your autonomic nervous system, which controls your fight-or-flight responses. When this system is balanced, you're better equipped to handle life's ups and downs without losing your cool.

So, what's the takeaway here? Breathwork isn't just about feeling good in the moment—it's a powerful tool for healing trauma and emotional well-being, supported by both personal experiences and science.

# Different Breathwork Techniques

Let's explore some techniques you can add to your healing toolkit, starting with the basics and moving toward more advanced practices. I promise to keep it light and easy to follow.

## *Diaphragmatic Breathing: Your Foundation for Healing*

Think of diaphragmatic breathing as the bread and butter of breathwork—simple, reliable, and oh-so-satisfying. This technique focuses on deep belly breaths, engaging your diaphragm, which sits right below your lungs.

Imagine your belly filling up like a balloon as you inhale and gently deflating as you exhale. It's all about calming the nervous system, a crucial piece of the trauma recovery puzzle.

Here's how to get started:

1. **Find a cozy place to settle in:** Either sit or recline in a location free from disturbances (yes, that includes silencing your phone).

2. **Rest a hand on your abdomen:** This helps you to sense its movement as you breathe.

3. **Breathe in deeply through your nose for a count of four:** Allow your belly to rise, not your chest.

4. **Exhale gently through your mouth for a count of six:** Softly push on your belly to release all the air.

5. **Continue this practice for five minutes:** Gradually extend the duration as you grow more comfortable.

This simple technique can be your go-to anytime you feel overwhelmed. Bonus: It's like giving your body a mini spa day; no appointment needed.

## *Boxed Breathing: Finding Your Rhythm*

Boxed breathing, or four-part breathing, is like the metronome for your breath—a steady, rhythmic pattern that brings calmness and control. Think of it as your secret weapon for managing anxiety when life gets extra messy.

Here's how to box breathe:

1. Breathe in through your nose for a count of four.

2. Pause your breath for another count of four. (Imagine it's like being submerged underwater—no need to stress, you've got this!)

3. Breathe out through your mouth for four counts.

4. Pause once more for four counts. Then, do it all over again.

It's simple, structured, and perfect for those moments when you need to regain control in the midst of chaos. Practice this for a few minutes each day, and you'll notice a sense of calm creeping in, even when life tries to test your patience.

## *Alternate Nostril Breathing: Balancing Mind and Body*

Alternate nostril breathing is like a brain massage—it soothes your mind while grounding your body. This technique involves—surprise!—breathing through alternate nostrils to balance your energy and emotions. It's great for trauma survivors who need to calm mental chatter and find emotional balance.

Here's how to try it:

1. Sit back and relax. Allow your left hand to rest gently in your lap while you bring your right hand up to your nose.

2. Use your thumb to close off your right nostril and take a deep breath in through your left nostril.

3. Next, use your ring finger to close your left nostril and breathe out through your right.

4. Inhale through your right nostril, then close it with your thumb and exhale through your left.

5. Continue this pattern for several minutes, alternating nostrils with each breath.

This might feel a little funny at first, but stick with it—it's worth the effort. You'll find yourself feeling more grounded and less caught up in the mental hamster wheel.

## *Clarity Breathwork: Emotional Release in Action*

Ready for a more advanced technique? Clarity breathwork takes things up a notch by integrating breath with emotional release. This practice involves continuous, connected breathing patterns that can help you unlock and release stored emotions.

Remember that shaken-up soda bottle? It is time to release some of that fizz.

Here's a step-by-step:

1. Create a comfortable setting. Seek out a serene location where you can recline and feel at ease.

2. Begin with rhythmic breathing. Inhale and exhale through your mouth in a seamless flow without any breaks in between.

3. Allow feelings to emerge. This is where the transformation occurs. As you breathe, you may sense emotions surfacing—embrace them. Cry, giggle, or even yell if necessary (try not to scare the dog).

4. Continue breathing for 15 to 20 minutes. Remain focused on your breath, accepting that whatever arises is part of your healing process.

5. Gradually return to your regular breathing. When you feel ready, slow down and let your breath find its natural pace again.

Clarity breathwork can be intense, so it's important to approach it with care. Make sure to hydrate, rest, and integrate whatever emotions come up after your session.

These techniques are here to support you as you continue your healing. Remember, nobody is aiming to be perfect during healing, just moving forward. Try each one, see what resonates with you, and make breathwork a regular part of your self-care routine. And hey, if all else fails, just remember to breathe. It's the simplest (and most underrated) tool in your healing toolbox.

# Guidelines for Practicing Breathwork

Breathwork can be one of the most powerful tools for healing, but like anything new, it requires a little preparation and patience. Let's look at some of the essentials, so you can integrate breathwork into your life in a way that feels natural and supportive. Whether you're new to this practice or looking to deepen your experience, let's walk through the key steps together.

### *Creating a Safe Space for Practice*

First—let's talk about your space. You don't need a Zen garden or a meditation room (though if you have them, fantastic!). All you need is a spot where you feel comfortable and can focus without distraction. Think of it as setting the stage for a moment with yourself. A calm, quiet space is important. This looks different for all of us. Are you most comfortable in your bed? Perfect! Are you at ease in a cozy chair in your living room? Wonderful. Are you most peaceful on your front porch? Amazing! Whatever feels like a sanctuary for you.

Now, let's add some personal touches. You might want to use essential oils (lavender for relaxation, anyone?), soft music, or your favorite blanket. These little details can help you feel safe and nurtured, which is vital when you're diving into emotional exploration. Remember, your space should invite you in and say, "Hey, it's okay to let go here."

And safety isn't just about the physical environment. Pay attention to your emotional safety as well. You're going to be exploring some deep waters with breathwork, so make sure you feel ready to dive in. Maybe that means having a supportive friend nearby or keeping a journal handy to capture any emotions that surface. Consider the timing too. It is likely not the best idea to dive into these waters if you are heading to a funeral that afternoon or meeting up with some toxic friends or family. Timing is everything.

## *Setting Your Intention*

Before you begin, ask yourself: *What do I want to release or heal today?* Setting an intention gives your breathwork purpose. It's like telling your body, "Okay, we're going to focus on this today, and I'm ready to let it go." Whether it's stress, an old emotional wound, or just the general tension of daily life, having a clear intention helps you direct your energy and breath toward that goal.

Think of your intention as the GPS for your breathwork road trip. Without it, you might still get somewhere, but with it, you're much more likely to end up exactly where you need to be. Take a moment to reflect on your emotional goals before starting. Are you looking to feel lighter? More connected to yourself? Whatever it is, hold that intention close as you breathe.

## *Consistency and Patience*

Here's the thing: breathwork isn't a one-and-done deal. It's a practice, which means it gets better with time and consistency. Healing takes time, and your progress might feel slow at times, but trust that every session is doing something powerful beneath the surface.

Be patient with yourself. There will be days when breathwork feels like wonderful and days when it feels like you're just sitting there breathing (which, let's be honest, we all are). Celebrate every day, like feeling a little lighter or more at peace. Over time, these small wins add up, and you'll start to notice big shifts in how you feel.

Do your best to remain consistent. Try to incorporate breathwork into your daily routine, even if it's just for a few minutes. Like brushing your teeth, it's the little daily habits that make the biggest difference over time.

## *Journaling and Reflection*

After your breathwork session, take a few minutes to journal about your experience. This doesn't have to be an epic novel; even just a few sentences about how you felt during and after the session can be insightful. Did any emotions come up? Did you notice any patterns or resistance? Journaling helps you track your progress and identify any barriers that might be standing in the way of your healing.

Reflection deepens your insights. When you choose to put your experiences into words, you make sense of them, and that's where the real growth happens. Plus, it's kind of amazing to look back after a few weeks or months and see how far you've come.

Your breathwork journal can become a powerful tool for self-discovery and healing.

## Final Thoughts

By now, you've got the tools to make breathwork a part of your life. You know how to create a safe space that invites healing, the importance of setting an intention, the value of consistency and patience, and the power of journaling and reflection. With these guidelines, you're ready to start—or continue—your breathwork journey, trusting that every breath brings you closer to releasing what no longer serves you and embracing the self-worth you deserve.

Let's get ready for the next chapter, where we will uncover the importance of mindfulness and meditation.

# Chapter 9:
# Mindfulness and Meditation

Does your mind ever feel like a cluttered closet, crammed with old emotions, stressful thoughts, and random worries that keep you up at 3:00 a.m. (like why you agreed to make your friend's birthday cake when you don't even own a cake pan)? Now, picture slowly opening that closet, not to shove more stuff in but to gently clear it out, piece by piece, until there's finally some breathing room.

In the upcoming pages, we'll talk about how mindfulness can help you catch those sneaky, self-critical thoughts before they spiral out of control and how meditation is like giving your brain a much-needed power nap. We'll laugh, learn, and discover that healing from within doesn't have to be difficult—it just needs a little bit of focus and a whole lot of kindness toward yourself.

## The Essence of Mindfulness

Imagine your mind as a party—thoughts coming in like guests, each with their own quirks, demands, and, of course, drama. Some are overenthusiastic, dancing wildly in the middle of the room (hello, anxious thoughts), while others sulk in a corner, refusing to leave (yes, you, lingering regrets). Mindfulness is like being the cool, calm host who acknowledges every guest but doesn't let any one of them take over the whole event.

## *Definition of Mindfulness*

At its core, mindfulness is the art of being present. It's that sweet spot where you're actively engaged in whatever you're doing without getting swept up in the chaos of your thoughts and emotions. Think of it as the mental equivalent of balancing on a tightrope—you're aware of everything around you, but you don't let anything throw you off balance.

Mindfulness allows us to observe our thoughts and feelings without judgment, which is key. It's like watching clouds pass by without chasing after them or trying to change their shape. In a healing context, this means noticing when old traumas or uncomfortable emotions arise, but instead of running from them (or screaming at them to get lost), you sit with them. This present-moment awareness helps you regulate your emotions better and brings a sense of peace.

## *Historical Context*

Mindfulness may feel like the latest buzzword, but it's actually been around for thousands of years, with roots in Buddhist traditions. Picture a serene monk seated under a tree, completely immersed in the now, contemplating the mysteries of the universe (and maybe wondering what's for lunch). The goal wasn't just to sit still—it was about connecting with the present moment to transcend the noise of daily life.

Fast forward to today, and mindfulness has evolved, popping up everywhere, from therapy sessions to corporate wellness programs. It's become a universal practice that transcends cultural boundaries, which means you don't have to shave your head or move to a monastery to get the benefits. You just need to show up—fully, wherever you are.

Understanding this history can deepen your appreciation for mindfulness, reminding you that it's more than just a trend. It's a practice that has helped people across centuries, and now it's your turn to experiment. Whether you start with mindful breathing, mindful eating, or even mindful dishwashing (yes, that's a thing), the key is finding what resonates with you. After all, it's not one-size-fits-all—it's about what fits you best.

## Mindfulness in Healing

Mindfulness is like shining a flashlight into the dark corners of your mind. It's about paying attention to what's happening right here, right now, without judging it. You might think, "Great, so I'll just sit with my thoughts and see what comes up. Easy, right?" Well, not always. Sometimes what pops up is a memory from third grade that you'd rather not think about (you know the one). Or maybe it's that nagging anxiety about the future that keeps looping in your head like a broken record. But here's the magic: By shining that flashlight on it, you're already starting to heal.

Mindfulness is a bridge—a sturdy one, not a rickety one with missing planks—that connects your present self with your past experiences. When you're mindful, you create a safe space to acknowledge that old trauma, the one that's been lurking in your subconscious like a bad movie villain. By being aware of it, you can start to process it. Think of mindfulness as inviting your trauma to sit down for a cup of tea instead of letting it hide in the attic making spooky noises.

For example, imagine you're Josh, the guy who used PSYCH-K to heal from losing his wife. One day, you're sitting at your kitchen table, and out of nowhere, you're hit with a wave of grief. But instead of shoving it down or distracting yourself, you decide to breathe deeply, acknowledge the pain, and be present with it. You're not trying to fix it or make it go away—you're just sitting with it, like an old friend who needs some time to be heard. This is mindfulness in action.

Mindfulness can significantly decrease anxiety and emotional distress. Why? Because it pulls you out of that endless loop of worrying about what could happen or ruminating on what already did. It brings you into the present moment, where you realize that right now, you're okay. That thought alone can feel like taking a deep breath after holding it for way too long.

Mindfulness empowers you to reclaim your personal narrative. When you sit with your emotions and experiences without judgment, you start to see them for what they are—just parts of your story, not the whole thing. You're no longer the helpless character trapped in a never-ending cycle of trauma. You become the author of your own story, choosing how to move forward.

Think of it like this: your trauma may have written some chapters in your life, but mindfulness hands you the pen to write the rest. And in those new chapters, you get to decide who you want to be. You get to reclaim your narrative, not by erasing the past, but by integrating it into your present with compassion and awareness.

So, next time you're feeling anxious or overwhelmed, try a simple mindfulness practice—take a few deep breaths, notice what's happening in your body and mind, and remind yourself that you are here now. You might find that this little practice helps you unlock your body's energy, release old trauma, and embrace your self-worth in a way that feels light-hearted, empowering, and—dare I say—kind of funny.

# Mindfulness Techniques

Let's explore mindfulness through the story of Patti—a woman who's been through the wringer but is still standing. Patti's life took a series of sharp left turns: she lost her job after 25 years, her husband of 30 years wanted out, and she took care of her mother through an 8-year battle with dementia. By the end of it all, Patti felt like a human deflated balloon—mentally and physically exhausted. Thankfully, she's been enjoying her weekly Reiki sessions, but now she's decided to give mindfulness a whirl.

## *Mindful Eating With Patti*

Patti starts with mindful eating because, well, food is life, right? Instead of scarfing down lunch while catching up on missed emails, she tries something new—eating one raisin. Yes, just one. At first, it feels a little ridiculous, but she gives it a go. She picks up the raisin and notices its texture: wrinkly, a little sticky, and definitely not the most glamorous fruit in the world. But then she smells it, feels it against her fingertips, and finally, after what feels like an eternity, pops it into her mouth.

This is where things get interesting. Instead of just chewing and swallowing, she lets the raisin sit on her tongue, noticing the sweetness, the slight tartness, and how her mouth naturally starts to produce saliva. She chews slowly, savoring every bit, and before she knows it, she's in a full-on Zen mode. For the first time in forever, Patti isn't thinking about bills, her next errand, or that endless to-do list. She's just... eating.

Mindful eating isn't about turning every meal into a slow-motion movie scene. It's about taking a few moments to truly taste and appreciate what's in front of you. Whether it's a raisin or a slice of pizza, slowing down allows you to be present, to breathe, and to give your mind a break from the usual chaos. Patti finds this little exercise surprisingly calming—and a nice break from her usual routine of eating while standing at the kitchen counter or in her car while doing errands.

## *Body Scan With Patti*

Next, Patti tries a body scan. It sounds fancy, but really, it's just a way to check in with your body, like giving yourself a mental massage. She lies down on her bed, closes her eyes, and starts at her toes. She notices they're a bit cold—probably should've worn those socks her daughter got her for Christmas. She wiggles them and moves her attention to her legs. Are they tense? A little, but nothing a good stretch won't fix.

As Patti mentally scans her body, she realizes she's been holding tension in her shoulders—no surprise there, given her stress load. Instead of getting frustrated, she takes a deep breath and lets her shoulders relax. She continues up to her neck (also tight, but again, not unexpected) and finally reaches her head. Patti realizes her face has been scrunched up in concentration, so she consciously relaxes her jaw and softens her forehead. By the end of the scan, she feels more at ease, like she just hit the refresh button on her body. She takes a few moments to lay, relaxed and loose. She isn't afraid to admit this has led to a nap on more than one occasion.

What Patti loves about these mindfulness exercises is how easy they are to incorporate into her daily life. She doesn't need any special equipment or a fancy meditation room. She can practice mindful eating at any meal, even if it's just savoring the first few bites. And body scans? Those can happen anywhere—before bed, during a break, or even in the middle of a hectic day when she just needs to reset.

By blending mindfulness into her routine, Patti feels more connected to herself, less frazzled, and a little more in control. And isn't that something we could all use a little more of?

# Benefits of Adopting Mindfulness

Mindfulness has become a bit of a buzzword these days, but what does it really offer? Let's break it down and show just how life-changing this practice can be.

## *Stress Reduction: Mindfulness as a Soothing Pause Button*

For the third day in a row, you find yourself sitting in a business meeting that just won't end. It is running late, and your stress is climbing as fast as your blood pressure. You feel your pulse in your temples, your hands gripping your coffee cup like it's the only thing keeping you from losing it completely. Enter mindfulness. Taking just a few deep breaths, you bring your attention to the present moment—letting go of the imagined smashing of said cup and walking out forever. Suddenly, you're aware of your surroundings—that bird outside the window; the warm feeling on your hands from the cup; your breath moving in and out—it's like hitting the pause button on chaos.

Studies even back this up, showing that mindfulness practices can lower cortisol (the stress hormone) levels in your body (Fincham et al., 2023). This means less wear and tear on your system and more resilience when life tests you.

## *Emotional Regulation: Becoming the Calm in Your Own Storm*

Let's talk emotions. Remember that time you got into an argument with your partner, and before you knew it, you were yelling over something completely unrelated to the actual issue? We have all been there. Maybe they had to reschedule a really important date, but within seconds, you found yourself screaming about dirty socks on the bedroom floor. That's what happens when emotions hijack us. Now, picture being able to hit pause during that moment of emotional overwhelm. Mindfulness invites us to notice our emotions instead of letting them drive the car.

Think of it like standing on the shore and watching waves roll in. Instead of getting pulled under by the tide of anger, frustration, or sadness, mindfulness allows you to stand firm and observe the waves. You see them coming, and they pass. Over time, this practice strengthens your emotional intelligence, allowing you to handle the highs and lows of life with more grace and fewer meltdowns.

How does this translate? "You know, I am really hurt about having to reschedule this date, but I understand your work meeting is important. Can we set a new date now so we have that to look forward to? On another note, I am going to need you to start picking up your socks so I can find peace in my life and not shave off your eyebrows while you sleep!" You get the picture, right?

## *Improved Focus and Clarity: Sharpening the Mind's Lens*

Ever had that moment when your brain feels like a computer with too many tabs open? Mindfulness can help you close some of those tabs. For instance, you're working on a project, but your mind keeps wandering to your grocery list, overdue bills, and that awkward conversation you had yesterday. Mindfulness helps you gently guide your attention back to the task at hand.

When you practice mindfulness, you train your brain to focus better, like turning the lens on a camera until the image is crystal clear. And with that clarity comes better decision-making and problem-solving. Suddenly, that looming project seems a little less looming, and you're able to tackle it with a sharper, more peaceful mind.

## *Enhanced Relationships: Showing Up Fully in Every Interaction*

Mindfulness isn't just about what's happening in your own head—it's about how you show up in your relationships, too. Let's say you're having a conversation with a friend, but instead of actively listening, you're already thinking about how to respond. Mindfulness invites you to be fully present, listening with intention and empathy, and not making it about you. I always suggest looking at this like, "How would I want this to look for me?" When you are talking to your friends, the more invested they are, the more important you feel. Be that friend.

Think of it as turning down the noise in your own mind so you can truly hear the other person. Over time, this practice can lead to healthier, more fulfilling relationships because you're no longer reacting on autopilot. You're responding thoughtfully, with a genuine understanding of the other person's perspective.

Incorporating mindfulness into your healing can be the key to unlocking a life of more peace, clarity, and connection—both with yourself and with others. Plus, it's way cheaper than therapy (though therapy is great, too!).

## Different Methods of Meditation

Meditation can feel like trying to catch a chicken with your bare hands at first—slippery and elusive. But once you get the hang of it, it becomes a daily ritual of peace. Here's a breakdown of different methods, so you can find what works best for you:

- **Guided meditation:** Imagine a wise friend holding your hand, leading you through a lush garden, pointing out all the hidden gems. That's guided meditation. These sessions, usually led by a soothing voice or a recording, help structure your experience, keeping your wandering mind on track. For beginners, this is a life-saver—no more sitting there wondering if you're "doing it right." Guided meditations cover everything from stress relief to confidence-building, so you can find something that speaks directly to your current needs. Think of it as having a meditation mentor in your pocket.

- **Mindfulness meditation:** Now, let's get a bit more DIY. Mindfulness meditation is all about tuning into the present moment—no bells, no whistles, just you and your breath. You focus on your breathing or do a body scan to create a bridge between mind and body. The goal? Simply noticing your thoughts without getting tangled up in them, like watching clouds drift by without chasing them.

Here's where we meet Dan. Dan, a project manager at a bustling tech company, used to be the guy who took on too much, overcommitted and then spiraled into stress-ville. His constant anxiety stemmed from a deep-seated belief that he wasn't good enough—a lovely little package from his childhood. Dan decided to try body scans (or progressive muscle relaxation—PMR for the initiated). At first, he felt ridiculous, lying there in bed, systematically relaxing his toes, then his calves, then his thighs. But soon enough, he noticed something: His anxiety wasn't as sharp, and his body was less tense. When he regularly tuned into himself, he started breaking the cycle of feeling unworthy, one muscle group at a time.

- **Visualization:** Ever daydream about winning an Oscar? Visualization is like that but with more purpose and less red carpet. This meditation technique lets you create vivid mental images that help you heal or manifest what you want. Picture yourself surrounded by healing light, or envision your future self, nailing that promotion or crossing a finish line. Visualization works because it taps into your emotional energy, linking your goals to powerful feelings, which can make them feel more real and achievable. It's like crafting your own movie, with you as the lead, always winning.

- **Loving-kindness meditation:** This one's all about the feels. Loving-kindness meditation involves sending warm, fuzzy vibes to yourself and others. Picture yourself handing out kindness like Oprah handing out cars: "You get love! And you get love! Everyone gets love!" Starting with yourself, you extend this good energy outward, even to that one person who cut you off in traffic last week. This practice is a self-worth booster and teaches you to approach tough emotions with a sense of compassion. It's like hugging your inner critic and telling them to take the day off.

Meditation doesn't have to be complicated or mystical. Whether you need guidance, a bit of mindfulness, the power of visualization, or the warmth of loving-kindness, there's a practice out there that fits your path. Experiment with these methods and see what helps unlock your body's energy, heal stored trauma, and embrace the self-worth you truly deserve.

# Practices to Integrate Mindfulness in Daily Life

Imagine that you've just had a heart attack. The very thing you always thought happened to *other* people. Suddenly, life as you knew it flips upside down, and fear wraps around you like a heavy blanket. That's the case with John, a 54-year-old man who had a heart attack a few months ago. Anxiety became his new companion, and he found himself caught in a cycle of worry, afraid of every twinge in his chest, every irregular breath.

His doctor suggested a lifestyle change, including mindfulness practices. John rolled his eyes at the suggestion. How was mindfulness supposed to stop him from having another heart attack? But after some gentle nudging, John reluctantly agreed to try mindful walking. It seemed simple enough—walking was something he could handle. And if it helped, well, why not?

## *Mindful Walking*

John started walking in his neighborhood park every morning. The first few days, he walked out of obligation, his mind still racing with worries about his heart. But then something changed. He began to notice the crunch of the gravel under his shoes, the cool breeze brushing his skin, the rhythmic sound of his own breath. Without realizing it, he had started synchronizing his breathing with his steps: inhale, step right; exhale, step left. The simplicity of it calmed his mind. He wasn't just walking anymore—he was *present*.

Day by day, as he practiced this mindful walking, John noticed a difference. His anxiety slowly started to loosen its grip. The movement, paired with his breath, created a sense of calm he hadn't felt in months. His body sensations became signals of life, not threats. The sounds of the park—birds chirping, leaves rustling—became comforting reminders that he was still here, still alive, still moving forward. His heart was healing, both physically and emotionally.

The results? John didn't just heal; he started to *thrive*. His morning walks became a routine he looked forward to, not just for his physical health but for his mental clarity. The mindfulness he fostered during these walks began to ripple into other areas of his life. He found himself more present during conversations, more patient with himself, and more at ease with his recovery.

## *Mindfulness Reminders: Nudging Yourself to Be Present*

But mindfulness doesn't have to be a dedicated time-consuming practice. The beauty of mindfulness lies in its flexibility—it can be blended into your day with just a few intentional cues. For John, it was small reminders throughout the day that helped him stay grounded. He set an hourly reminder on his phone that simply read, "Breathe." Every time his phone buzzed, he paused, took a deep breath, and just *noticed* his surroundings. Those small moments of mindfulness helped him reconnect to his body and calm his mind, even on the busiest days.

You can set up these reminders, too. Visual cues like sticky notes on your bathroom mirror that say, "Be here now," or auditory nudges like a gentle chime on your phone can prompt you to pause for a moment. You can even practice "habit stacking" by pairing mindfulness with existing routines—take a few mindful breaths while brushing your teeth or focus on your senses while washing the dishes. These simple strategies make mindfulness accessible, no matter how hectic your day might be.

### *Journaling: Writing Your Way to Mindfulness*

If you're someone who processes through writing, journaling can be a powerful mindfulness practice. For John, journaling became his evening ritual—a way to reflect on his day, organize his thoughts, and let go of the lingering worries. He found that by writing about his experiences, he could gain a deeper understanding of his anxiety and gradually release the fears that were still holding him back.

Journaling doesn't have to be complex. Start with simple prompts like, "What did I notice today?" or "How did I feel during my mindful walk?" This reflective writing can help you solidify your mindfulness practice, giving you a space to process emotions and validate your experiences. Over time, you may find that journaling becomes a therapeutic tool for emotional release, allowing you to fully embrace your healing.

# Final Thoughts

By integrating mindfulness into your daily life through practices like mindful walking, mindful eating, reminders, and journaling, you're equipping yourself with tools to build your awareness and healing. These strategies are simple yet powerful, allowing you to reconnect with your body, manage stress, and foster a deeper sense of peace.

It is time to move into the final chapter. Here we will discover supportive habits and practices for ongoing emotional health and well-being.

# Chapter 10:
# Supportive Habits and Practices

You've made it to the final chapter! You've done the work, peeled back the layers, and unlocked some seriously powerful energy within you. So now what? How do you keep that spark going, even on days when life feels more like a never-ending laundry cycle than a spiritual awakening?

This chapter is your toolkit for maintaining the good energy long after you've turned the last page. Think of it as your self-care maintenance plan. We're talking about real-life, down-to-earth practices that will help you stay grounded and clear, like the emotional equivalent of making sure your phone battery doesn't dip below 5%. (Because, let's face it, nobody wants to be in low-power mode.)

## Creating a Sleep Routine

Creating a sleep routine might sound like a no-brainer, but it's one of the most powerful—and often overlooked—ways to help your body and mind heal from trauma.

When you think about it, sleep is your body's nightly reboot, and we all know how irritable our tech gets when we skip a reboot. Imagine how much better we'd feel if we treated ourselves to a regular, peaceful reboot every night!

## *Importance of Sleep Hygiene*

Think of sleep hygiene as your nighttime toolkit for better emotional health. It's not just about avoiding coffee before bed (though, yeah, that's a biggie), but about building a routine that tells your body, "Hey, it's time to unwind." Having a consistent sleep schedule is like setting your internal alarm clock on a nice, predictable timer. It helps your body understand when it's time to sleep and when it's time to wake up.

So, what does a good sleep schedule look like? This doesn't have to get complicated. Going to bed and waking up at the same time every day (yes, even on weekends) helps keep that internal clock ticking smoothly. Your body thrives on consistency, and when you give it a reliable rhythm, your mood, energy, and resilience naturally follow suit.

Creating a peaceful sleep environment is another biggie. If your bedroom is a cluttered mess, your brain is going to be a cluttered mess too. Tidy it up, ditch the harsh lights, and add some calming scents—think lavender or chamomile. It's like making your bed a sanctuary, a place where stress isn't invited. You should actually get excited about climbing into your bed. Spend time picking out a comfortable mattress and cozy bedding. Don't forget to consider the temperature in your room. Keeping it cooler while you sleep will keep you cozy and sleeping better longer.

## *Techniques for Better Sleep*

So, how do we actually make sleep better? First off, herbal teas and breathing exercises can become your new best friends. Sipping on a warm cup of chamomile tea or practicing deep breathing you've learned in this book before bed signals to your body that it's time to switch gears. It's like sending out an invitation to your brain, saying, "Let's chill out, shall we?"

Now, about those screens. I know, I know, scrolling through social media right before bed is practically a national pastime, but limiting screen time can do wonders for your sleep. The blue light from screens tricks your brain into thinking it's still daytime, which is the exact opposite of what you want before bed. Try swapping your phone for a book or some calming music instead. Consider listening to a calming, peaceful audiobook.

And here's a pro tip: Keep a sleep journal. It's not just for insomniacs; it's for anyone who wants to understand their sleep patterns better. In your journal, jot down things like what time you went to bed, how long it took you to fall asleep, and how rested you feel in the morning. It can help you spot patterns and figure out what's affecting your sleep quality. Here's a little exercise: Start your journal tonight, and write about what you did before bed, how long you slept, and how you felt in the morning. After a week, look for trends—what's working and what's not?

## *Addressing Sleep Issues*

Insomnia is no joke; if you're dealing with it, you're not alone. Trauma often has a way of sneaking into our sleep, making it hard to rest. But the first step in healing is acknowledging that insomnia might be rooted in unresolved trauma. This awareness doesn't just make sleep issues feel less like a personal failure; it gives you a starting point for healing.

If sleep issues are keeping you up, try adaptive strategies to turn those struggles into opportunities for self-care. For example, mindfulness and relaxation techniques like deep breathing, journaling, and meditation can calm an overactive mind. Deep breathing slows down your heart rate, journaling helps release those pesky thoughts swirling in your head, and meditation guides you into a peaceful state of mind.

### *Establishing Calming Pre-Sleep Rituals*

Let's talk about winding down. Creating calming rituals before bed helps bridge the gap between your busy day and restful sleep. This could be something as simple as gentle yoga or stretching, which not only relaxes your muscles but also calms your mind. Try a few light stretches or a short yoga sequence before bed—it's like giving your body a gentle "goodnight."

Another great practice is writing gratitude lists. Shift your focus from the stresses of the day to the things you're thankful for. It might sound simple, but ending your day with positive thoughts can actually make you feel more at ease as you drift off to sleep.

Sleep isn't just sleep—it's one of the most important pillars of emotional and physical health. When you implement restorative routines and create your own personal sleep sanctuary, you're setting the foundation for deeper healing. Start by focusing on consistent schedules, calming pre-sleep rituals, and adapting strategies to manage sleep disturbances. With these simple steps, you'll be on your way to better emotional resilience and self-worth, one peaceful night at a time.

# Reducing Stress Effectively

Reducing stress effectively isn't about avoiding stress altogether (because, let's be real, life is stressful). Instead, it's about having the right tools to face stress head-on and managing it before it morphs into something that eats away at your emotional and physical health. Think of it like this: You wouldn't expect to cook dinner without any ingredients, right? Stress management is the same. Let's fill up your stress-relief toolbox, so you're always prepared for life's wild ride.

## *Understanding Stress: The Body-Mind Tango*

Stress is sneaky—it doesn't just hit you in the head; it takes over your whole body. Ever notice how your shoulders creep up to your ears when you're tense? Or how your stomach feels like it's hosting a boxing match? That's stress manifesting physically, especially if you're already dealing with trauma. It's like trauma's annoying friend that shows up uninvited, bringing headaches, stomach aches, and a racing heart to the party.

Recognizing your stress triggers is key. Maybe it's a jam-packed schedule, an impending deadline, or just the sound of your alarm clock (why do they always sound so aggressive?). Knowing what sets you off helps you hit the pause button before stress turns into a full-on meltdown. Plus, when you understand how your body responds to stress—whether it's clammy hands, rapid breathing, or the sudden urge to flee—you're in a better position to manage it effectively.

## *Mind-Body Techniques: Instant Calm Hacks*

When stress hits, you need quick, practical strategies. Enter the mind-body connection: your secret weapon for instant calm.

- **Deep breathing sessions:** When your brain is running a mile a minute, and your to-do list feels endless, it's time to hit the pause button. Deep breathing is your go-to tool for instant relief. Here's how it works: close your eyes, take a deep breath in through your nose for a count of four, hold it for another four, and then exhale slowly through your mouth for four. It's like giving your brain a mini vacation—just in a few seconds. As you breathe deeply, you're signaling to your nervous system that it's okay to relax. Suddenly, that mountain of stress feels more like a molehill. The beauty of deep breathing is that you can do it anytime, anywhere. Whether you're in the middle of a hectic day or just trying to unwind before bed, a few deep breaths can reset your mind and body, leaving you feeling calm and in control.

- **Visualization techniques:** Ever find yourself wishing for an escape button when life gets too intense? Visualization is like teleporting to your personal paradise without leaving your chair. Close your eyes and let your imagination take the lead—whether you're envisioning the soothing waves of a beach, the crisp air of a mountain peak, or the cozy comfort of your own bed. The key is to make it as real as possible. Imagine the details: the warmth of the sun on your skin, the sound of the waves, the scent of pine trees, or the softness of your favorite blanket. This mental escape tricks your brain into feeling calm and peaceful, even when you're knee-deep in deadlines or dealing with a less-than-pleasant situation. Visualization is your secret weapon for instant serenity, no matter where you are or what you're facing.

- **Grounding exercises:** When stress makes you feel like you're floating away in a storm of thoughts and emotions, grounding exercises are the anchor that pulls you back to solid ground. It's all about reconnecting with the present moment and your physical surroundings. Start by focusing on what's around you: what can you see, hear, or touch right now? Feel the weight of your body as your feet press firmly against the ground. Wiggle your toes if you need to remind yourself that you're here, rooted in the present. Grounding exercises help you break free from the whirlwind of stress and remind you that, in this moment, you are safe, you are steady, and you are in control. It's like a reality check for your senses, bringing you back to where you are and giving you the clarity to face whatever comes next.

## *Creating a Personal Stress-Relief Toolbox: Your Custom Kit*

Let's talk tools—not the hammer-and-nails kind, but your personal stress-relief toolkit. The key here is personalization—what works for you might not work for someone else, and that's okay. You're unique, after all.

Start by identifying your strengths. Are you a creative soul who feels better after some crafty time? Or do you prefer physical activities like yoga or dancing? Journaling can also be a great release, especially if you enjoy putting pen to paper and letting your thoughts spill out.

The magic happens when you build variety into your stress-relief kit. Maybe some days you need a good workout to blow off steam, and other days, a quiet moment of meditation is all it takes. Keep your options open so that you're ready for whatever stress throws your way.

Take a moment to write out your favorite stress-busting activities. These can be anything from painting to walking your dog or even just sipping tea in silence.

Think of things that bring a smile to your face, keep you relaxed, and make you happy and relaxed.

_____
_____
_____
_____
_____
_____
_____

Now, group these activities into categories like "quick fixes" (deep breathing, stretching), "creative outlets" (journaling, drawing), and "physical activities" (walking, yoga). Voilà—your personalized stress-relief toolbox!

| Quick Fixes | Creative Outlets | Physical Activities |
|---|---|---|
|  |  |  |
|  |  |  |
|  |  |  |
|  |  |  |
|  |  |  |

## *Setting Boundaries: The Power of "No"*

Be mindful that you only have so much energy, and it's okay to protect it. Saying "no" is an act of self-care, even if it feels uncomfortable at first. When you acknowledge your limits, you're respecting yourself, which is important for maintaining your emotional health.

Think of it like refueling your car. You wouldn't keep driving on empty, right? The same goes for your personal energy levels. Setting boundaries means empowering yourself to step back when needed and preventing emotional fatigue before it wipes you out completely. Remind yourself that it is okay to delegate and ask for help, you don't have to do everything on your own.

And don't forget, setting boundaries isn't just for your benefit—it's also about nurturing healthier relationships. When you clearly communicate your limits, you're showing others how to respect your needs while maintaining your self-worth. It's a win for everyone!

Stress is inevitable, but how you handle it is in your hands. Mastering these stress management techniques allows you to build a resilient mindset that empowers you to tackle life's challenges with grace, humor, and a sense of calm. Remember, your body's energy is your most precious resource—protect it, and it will protect you right back.

# Incorporating Proper Nutrition and Exercise

When we think about unlocking the body's energy to release trauma and welcome self-worth, nutrition and exercise might sound like that boring pair of shoes in your closet you know you should wear but avoid for the fun sneakers instead.

But let's break it down into something more relatable—less "Eat your veggies!" and more "How can I feel good without feeling deprived?"

## *Nutrition for Mental Health: Food That Feeds Your Feel-Good Energy*

Imagine your brain is like a garden. What you feed it either helps it bloom or lets weeds take over. The connection between food and mood is real, and understanding it can be like finding out that chocolate is indeed part of a balanced diet (okay, maybe not, but bear with me).

You know those days when you just feel off? Sometimes, it's not just the stress from work or a tough conversation; it could also be the food you've been putting into your body. Nutrient-rich foods, like colorful fruits, vegetables, and whole grains, have the power to increase your cognitive functions, giving you mental clarity that might feel like that first sip of coffee in the morning—only without the jitters.

Now, let's talk about omega-3 fatty acids. You might be wondering, "Are those the fish oil capsules my grandma keeps raving about?" Yes! These little wonders are linked to lower levels of depression. So, if you're thinking of skipping the salmon at dinner, you might want to reconsider—your brain will thank you. And let's not forget the joy of eating whole foods with others. Sharing meals isn't just about food; it's about connection, which can be incredibly healing. Imagine a potluck where everyone brings something wholesome and delicious—it's like a community therapy session, only tastier.

## Creating Balanced Meals: Ditch the Guilt and Love Your Plate

Speaking of meals, let's get real—meal prep can feel like a second job. But think of it as self-care in disguise. When you prepare balanced meals ahead of time, you reduce that midweek "What's for dinner?" panic when takeout ends up being the answer.

Start simple: plan a few meals that you genuinely enjoy and can easily prepare. Think of it as building a relationship with your future self—one that says, "Hey, I got your back, and yes, there's lasagna waiting for you after that long day."

Portion sizes are another thing. If you're like me, you've gone from all-in on a strict diet to eating pizza straight out of the box in a single sitting. The key is balance—finding portions that satisfy you without triggering the guilt that often follows overindulgence. And remember, setting realistic dietary goals is like planting seeds that will actually grow over time. Fad diets are like trying to grow a palm tree in the desert—not sustainable and pretty frustrating.

## Integrating Movement Into Daily Life

Now, exercise doesn't have to mean signing up for that intense boot camp before the sun rises (unless that's your thing—more power to you!). The secret is finding movement that feels good and sneaking it into your day. Did you know that even short bursts of activity can make a difference? Think of it like stacking wins—each bit of movement adds up to something bigger.

Not a fan of traditional exercise? No problem. Maybe dancing around your living room to your favorite playlist or walking with a friend could be your thing. The goal here is to find joy in movement, turning it into a regular part of life rather than a dreaded chore. And the best part? Movement isn't just good for your body; it also balances your emotions. Ever had one of those days when you felt better just by getting outside for fresh air? It's like nature's gift to you.

Your body is an ecosystem, and when you feed it well and keep it moving, you're doing yourself a benefit. The right foods and enjoyable physical activities can help you build emotional resilience, making it easier to handle whatever life throws your way. And who wouldn't want that?

## Fostering Healthy Relationships

Healthy relationships are the cornerstone of emotional healing and self-worth. Once you are able to recognize toxic patterns, build supportive networks, practice effective communication, and welcome vulnerability, you can foster connections that nurture your emotional health. Here's how to unlock your body's energy to release trauma and embrace self-worth through the relationships in your life.

- **Recognizing toxic patterns:** Ever felt like your energy was being sucked right out of you after hanging out with certain people? It's like they're emotional vampires—without the cool cape. These are the people who drain your energy and make you question your self-worth. Recognizing these toxic patterns is the first step to reclaiming your emotional health. If every time you interact with someone, you leave feeling worse, that's a sign. Reflect on these relationships. Do they build you up or tear you down? Sometimes, the healthiest choice is to take a step back. It's like giving your garden a chance to grow by pulling out the weeds.

- **Building supportive networks:** Imagine surrounding yourself with people who make you feel like the sun is shining, even on a cloudy day. That's the goal—cultivating a network of supportive, energizing influences that feed your soul. Whether it's a friend who makes you laugh until your stomach hurts or a mentor who always knows the right thing to say, these are the connections that will help you heal and thrive. Engaging in community activities, whether it's a book club, a yoga class, or volunteering, is another way to meet positive influences. It's like planting new seeds that will grow into a supportive network of people who've got your back.

- **Effective communication skills:** Now, let's talk communication. Think of it as the water your garden needs to thrive. Practicing active listening—where you really hear what the other person is saying, not just waiting for your turn to talk—helps deepen connections. It's like pouring water on those new seedlings, giving them a chance to grow strong roots. Using "I" statements, such as "I feel…" instead of "You always…," can make a world of difference. It lowers defenses and creates a safe space for honest conversations. And setting up regular check-ins with loved ones is like scheduling time to tend to your garden, making sure everything stays healthy and connected.

- **Embracing vulnerability:** Finally, there's vulnerability. I know it sounds scary, but it's more like fertilizer for your emotional garden. Being open about your struggles allows trust to grow. When you share, you invite others to share, too, creating deeper connections. Vulnerability isn't weakness; it's strength. It's the thing that makes your garden thrive. Welcoming vulnerability, you cultivate relationships grounded in empathy and mutual support—like a garden that blooms with the help of every plant around it.

It is time to start tending to your garden of relationships today and watch as you flourish right alongside it.

## Final Thoughts

As we wrap up this time together, imagine your supportive habits and practices as a toolkit, but not the rusty, old kind you keep in the garage. Think of it as a bright, shiny box filled with the best tools for your well-being, all designed to help you unlock your body's energy and embrace your worth. You've already been doing the hard work of releasing trauma, like finally letting go of that heavy suitcase you've been dragging through every airport of life. Now, it's time to fill that space with lighter, more helpful habits.

These tools won't fix everything overnight—that's not how this works. But they're here to support you, nudge you in the right direction, and remind you that you're worthy of every ounce of energy you put into yourself. So, keep them close, use them often, and know that every small step forward is a victory worth celebrating. After all, you're not just healing; you're growing into the most vibrant, powerful version of you. And that is worth holding onto.

# Chapter 11:
# Modality Chart

To help you keep track, we've included a simple chart that you can use to weigh the pros and cons of each energy healing modality we've explored in this book. Think of it as your personal scorecard—a place to jot down what worked, what didn't, and how each practice made you feel. Whether you're a fan of Reiki's gentle touch or found polarity therapy to be your go-to, this chart will help you reflect on your experiences. It's an easy way to see what's bringing you the most benefit, helping you make informed choices as you continue to unlock your body's energy and embrace your self-worth.

| Modality | Pros | Cons |
|---|---|---|
| EFT Tapping | | |
| PSYCH-K | | |
| Reiki | | |
| Somatic experiences | | |
| Polarity therapy | | |
| Breathwork | | |
| Mindfulness | | |
| Meditation | | |

# Conclusion

Throughout this book, we've walked together through the wild and wonderful intricacies of the mind-body connection. In *Oops, I've Packed My Trauma*, we've unveiled how trauma is tucked away in our bodies like that pesky dust under your bed, out of sight but definitely not out of mind. We explored many energy healing modalities, including EFT Tapping and Reiki, which might have sounded a bit "out there" at first, but as you now know, they're actually practical tools to help kickstart your healing journey.

We started by looking at how traumas, big or small, get lodged in our physical selves. Remember that time you stubbed your toe and swore the universe was out to get you? Well, imagine that on an emotional scale, where those little (or not so little) moments stick around and cause all kinds of havoc. But here's where we got proactive: With EFT tapping, we tapped away stress and those emotional roadblocks. It wasn't magic—although it felt magical when you realized how much lighter you felt afterward.

Reiki brought a whole new level of serenity. Hands-on or hands-off, who knew channeling life force energy could make such a difference? It's like having a reset button on your emotional hard drive. And remember our good friend mindfulness? That practice where focusing on your breath makes everything feel a tad more manageable and your grocery store meltdowns fewer?

Now, armed with these insights and tools, what's next? Remember that knowledge is power, but only if you use it. Take some time and reflect on the chart offered in the final chapter.

Each of the modalities offered in the book will work differently for each person. Review what worked and felt best for you.

Take what you've learned and start integrating the practices you choose into your everyday life. Have patience with yourself. Every time you pause to breathe deeply instead of reacting, every time you tap through a rough emotion, you're stepping closer to who you're meant to be without the baggage of stored trauma. Celebrate the progress you make because this is a testament to your commitment and courage.

Feel free to picture a future where the weight of past traumas no longer drags you down like a stubborn anchor. Imagine waking up feeling energized and excited about life, free from the invisible chains of old hurts. You find joy in the little things again; laughter isn't just an escape but a genuine expression of how light you feel. Relationships deepen as you connect with others from a place of wholeness rather than woundedness. And let's face it, your body might even thank you with less tension, fewer aches, and a spring in your step you thought was only for kids and kangaroos.

It's entirely within your reach to step into this brighter, healed version of yourself. The practices detailed in this book are not just exercises—they're pathways to a more empowered way of living. I encourage you to actively engage with your energy field, explore these healing techniques, and watch as your emotional, mental, and physical well-being flourish.

Before we part ways, I want to ask for something small but powerful: sharing your story. If "Oops, I've Packed My Trauma" has given you clarity or sparked a glimmer of hope, consider leaving a review. Your words could be the very encouragement someone else needs to start their own healing quest. If you share your experiences, you could create ripples of empowerment that can touch countless lives.

Plus, it's a great way to stay involved in a community of like-minded warriors working toward healing and growth.

So here we are at the end, but really, it's just the beginning. Take a moment to pat yourself on the back for making it through these pages—your curiosity and openness have led you here. Now, take that same spirit and apply it to your daily life. Embrace the wonderful world of energy healing. Keep exploring, keep practicing, and most importantly, keep believing in your capacity to heal.

Remember, each breath, each tap, each mindful moment is tied to a larger collective effort of people striving for betterment. Together, we make the world a little lighter, a little brighter, and a whole lot more joyful.

# Bonus Resources

To thank you for purchasing this book, we're offering a **FREE** journal! Though we've provided space within these pages to sort out what's on your mind, we understand that you might need a little more room to put down your thoughts and experiences as you work through each of the modalities.

Simply scan the QR code above or visit https://www.inner-spark.info/bonus#product to download your copy and continue along your energy healing journey.

To receive your **FREE** gift, you will be prompted to provide your name and email address. Please be sure to whitelist our email address violet@inner-spark.info so this valuable resource doesn't end up in your spam folder!

# Please Leave Us a Review

★★★★★

Thanks for purchasing this book. If this guide has provided you with valuable insights and practical applications, I'd love to hear from you!

Simply scan the QR code above or https://www.inner-spark.info/oops-i-packed-my-trauma and leave your feedback to help others who are seeking energy healing find the tools they need to succeed.

# Glossary

**Affirmations:** Positive statements you repeat to yourself, like "I am enough," even when the mirror reflects bedhead and smudged mascara. Affirmations help train your brain to believe good things about yourself, much like telling a dog they're a "good boy" over and over until they wag their tail with confidence.

**Breathwork:** Controlled breathing exercises that help manage emotions, reduce stress, and clear your mind. Imagine you're inflating a balloon with each breath, and with every exhale, you let go of the stress from that awkward Zoom meeting. It's like rebooting your nervous system, one breath at a time.

**Body scan meditation:** A mindfulness practice where you mentally "scan" your body from head to toe, noticing sensations without judgment. Think of it as an internal check-up—like when you slowly assess which part of your body hurts after a workout. Except here, you're doing it to release tension, not to curse at your trainer.

**EFT (Emotional Freedom Technique) tapping:** A method of tapping on specific meridian points on your body while repeating affirmations to release negative emotions. Picture yourself tapping on your forehead like a human stress eraser, and suddenly, that annoying comment from earlier feels less important.

**Energy healing:** Various techniques, such as Reiki or polarity therapy, that involve channeling energy to promote physical, emotional, and spiritual healing. Think of energy healing as charging your inner battery—no USB port required—just a practitioner with some good vibes and a healing touch.

**Energy fields:** Imagine the invisible Wi-Fi signals connecting your body to the universe. That's what energy fields are—vibrational forces that keep everything in sync, from your thoughts to your toe taps.

**Intention setting:** The practice of defining your goals and desires with clarity and purpose. It's like planting seeds in a garden; setting intentions is deciding what you want to grow in your life. Whether it's inner peace or a new habit, setting an intention gives you a road map to get there—just like making that to-do list on Sunday night.

**Meditation:** A practice of calming the mind, often by focusing on your breath or a mantra. It's like hitting the mute button on your thoughts, allowing you to find some peace in the chaos. Remember that moment when you just sat still and stared at the sunset, completely in the moment? That's meditation without even trying.

**Mindfulness:** The art of being fully present in the moment without letting your mind wander to the grocery list or that awkward thing you said at the party. Mindfulness helps you appreciate the little things, like the smell of fresh coffee or the warmth of the sun on your skin. It's like living life with all five senses turned on.

**Polarity therapy:** An energy healing practice that balances the body's energy fields to promote overall wellness. Picture your body as a tangled set of earbuds that Polarity Therapy helps untangle so everything flows smoothly again. It's like organizing your closet and suddenly finding it easier to get dressed in the morning—except this is organizing your energy.

**PSYCH-K:** A simple, effective method for reprogramming limiting subconscious beliefs. It's like upgrading your mental software so you're no longer operating on old, outdated beliefs. Remember when you finally updated your phone's operating system, and suddenly everything ran smoother? That's PSYCH-K for your mind.

**Progressive muscle relaxation:** A technique where you tense and then relax each muscle group in your body to release tension. It's like squeezing a stress ball really hard and then feeling that sweet relief when you let go. This practice reminds your body what it feels like to relax—even when life's throwing lemons at you.

**Reiki:** A Japanese energy healing technique where a practitioner channels healing energy into your body through light touch. Picture yourself as a phone on low battery, and Reiki is the universal charger that helps restore your energy levels. After a session, you might feel as refreshed as you do after a long nap on a lazy Sunday.

**Somatic experiencing:** A body-centered approach to healing trauma that focuses on releasing stored tension and stress in your body. Imagine you're a soda bottle that's been shaken up; Somatic Experiencing helps you open that bottle slowly and release the pressure without exploding. It's like feeling the knots in your shoulders untangle after a really good stretch.

**Visualization:** Visualization is like daydreaming on purpose. You close your eyes and picture something positive, like a beach or your favorite dessert, to help your body and mind get on the same happy page.

# Resources

- **eftinternational.org/discover-eft-tapping/what-is-eft-tapping:** The official website of the world's leading EFT professional organization. Here, you will find information on where to find practitioners, a free downloadable tapping point chart, and a how-to tap guide.

- **psych-k.com/about/:** The official website features information about PYSCH K, instructors, workshops, testimonials, frequently asked questions, and more.

- **youtu.be/6VDRqLNiSlQ:** Bruce Lipton's PSYCH-K introduction

- **digitaldrstone.org:** All of Dr. Randolph Stone's books on polarity therapy can be accessed for free here.

- **www.freemindfulness.org/download:** This is a great resource of free mindfulness and meditation exercises for you to download and use.

- **reikirays.com/reiki-resources-hub/:** This complete Reiki resource is filled with instructions on how to find the perfect practitioner and questions to ask.

- **traumahealing.org/resources/:** Straight from the Somatic Experience Institute, this resource has it all. You can find podcasts, videos, tutorials, books, and so much more.

- **soulbody.co/blog/get-started-with-breathwork:** A wonderful resource for breathwork. Here, you will find many exercises and tutorials at your fingertips.

- **breathlessexpeditions.com/the-best-breathwork-apps-this-year/:** Feel free to visit this site and explore the 12 best breathwork apps available to you. Read through the options and discover what each offers and which one is best suited for you.

- **norwestwellbeing.com.au/types-of-psych-k-balances/ and thevortex.me/stress-release/:** These are both great pages with supplemental PSYCH-K balance exercises.

- **youtube.com/watch?v=Ljss_Ut5pxY:** If you are looking for a self-guided EMDR session, this one is easy to follow.

# References

Ackerman, C. (2019, June 19). *What is self-concept theory? A psychologist explains.* Positive Psychology.com. https://positivepsychology.com/self-concept/

Anthony, K. (2023, April 6). *EFT tapping.* Healthline Media. https://www.healthline.com/health/eft-tapping

Bach, D., Groesbeck, G., Stapleton, P., Sims, R., Blickheuser, K., & Church, D. (2019). Clinical EFT (emotional freedom techniques) improves multiple physiological markers of health. *Journal of Evidence-Based Integrative Medicine*, *24*(24), 2515690X18823691. https://doi.org/10.1177/2515690X18823691

Banushi, B., Brendle, M., Ragnhildstveit, A., Murphy, T., Moore, C., Egberts, J., & Robison, R. (2023). Breathwork interventions for adults with clinically diagnosed anxiety disorders: A scoping review. *Brain Sciences*, *13*(2), 256. https://doi.org/10.3390/brainsci13020256

Baskin, J. (2024, March 25). *Road among tall trees in valley of the giants in oregon in USA* [Image]. Pexels. https://www.pexels.com/photo/road-among-tall-trees-in-valley-of-the-giants-in-oregon-in-usa-20762934/

*The benefits of reiki massage for stress relief and healing.* (2024, August 22). Kaizen Health Group.

https://kaizenhealthgroup.com/the-benefits-of-reiki-massage-for-stress-relief-and-healing/

Bremner, J. D. (2006). Traumatic stress: effects on the brain. *Dialogues in Clinical Neuroscience*, *8*(4), 445–461. https://www.ncbi.nlm.nih.gov/pmc/articles/PMC3181836/

Chhabra, G., & Prasad, A. (2019). Comparison and performance evaluation of human bio-field visualization algorithm. *Research Gate*, 1–12. https://doi.org/10.1080/13813455.2019.1680699

Chu, K.-H., Tung, H.-H., Clinciu, D. L., Hsu, H.-I., Wu, Y.-C., Hsu, C.-I., Lin, S.-W., & Pan, S.-J. (2022). A preliminary study on self-healing and self-health management in older adults: Perspectives from healthcare professionals and older adults in taiwan. *Gerontology and Geriatric Medicine*, *8*, 233372142210777. https://doi.org/10.1177/23337214221077788

Church, D., Stapleton, P., Mollon, P., Feinstein, D., Boath, E., Mackay, D., & Sims, R. (2018). Guidelines for the treatment of PTSD using clinical EFT (emotional freedom techniques). *Healthcare*, *6*(4). https://doi.org/10.3390/healthcare6040146

Church, D., Yount, G., & Brooks, A. J. (2012). The effect of emotional freedom techniques on stress biochemistry.

*Journal of Nervous & Mental Disease, 200*(10), 891–896. https://doi.org/10.1097/nmd.0b013e31826b9fc1

Cleveland Clinic. (2024, July 16). *What is reiki, and does it really work?* Cleveland Clinic. https://health.clevelandclinic.org/reiki

Cronkleton, E. (2018, June 22). *5 reasons you should try reiki.* Healthline. https://www.healthline.com/health/reiki

Cronkleton, E., & Walters, O. (2022, March 16). *Alternate nostril breathing: Benefits, how to, and more.* Healthline. https://www.healthline.com/health/alternate-nostril-breathing

Davis, S. (2022, May 9). *Chronic stress vs. complex trauma.* CPTSD Foundation. https://cptsdfoundation.org/2022/05/09/chronic-stress-vs-complex-trauma/

Demir Doğan, M. (2018). The effect of reiki on pain: A meta-analysis. *Complementary Therapies in Clinical Practice, 31,* 384–387. https://doi.org/10.1016/j.ctcp.2018.02.020

Dharma-Devi, D. (2022, March 24). *Clarity breathwork.* Dana Dharma Devi. https://clarity.org/clarity-breathwork/

EFT and polyvagal theory. (2022, May 10). *Eft and Mindfulness.* https://www.eftandmindfulness.com/blog/eft-and-the-vagus-nerve-polyvagal-theory

*EFT tapping points: 12 primary meridian points tapping.* (2023, February 11). Virtual Living College.

https://vitalitylivingcollege.info/eft-tapping-meridian-points/

*Expert training accelerates your mastery*. (2024, January 30). EFT Universe. https://eftuniverse.com/certification/the-eft-seminar/?gad_source=1&gclid=Cj0KCQjwzva1BhD3 ARIsADQuPnUrcd6BZVE3iy6EgPEOi8hULKeTlvsQ nLpHl8TubyQv5jLJl7wDjf4aAtl5EALw_wcB

Fannin, J., & Williams, R. (2011). QEEG reveals interactive link between the principles of business, the principles of nature and the whole-brain state . *NeuroConnections*. https://psych-k.com/wp-content/uploads/2013/10/neuroConnectionsV7-copy.pdf

Feinstein, D. (2023). Using energy psychology to remediate emotional wounds rooted in childhood trauma: preliminary clinical guidelines. *Frontiers*, *14*. https://doi.org/doi.org/10.3389/fpsyg.2023.1277555

Fincham, G. W., Mavor, K., & Dritschel, B. (2023). Effects of mindfulness meditation duration and type on well-being: An online dose-ranging randomized controlled trial. *Mindfulness*. https://doi.org/10.1007/s12671-023-02119-2

*5 kinds of somatic therapy*. (2022, April 18). Somatic Psychotherapy in New York City.

https://www.downtownsomatictherapy.com/article/5-kinds-of-somatic-therapies

Fraley, C. (2019). *Your personality*. Yourpersonality.net. https://yourpersonality.net/attachment/

Gautam, S., Jain, A., Chaudhary, J., Gautam, M., Gaur, M., & Grover, S. (2024). Concept of mental health and mental well-being, it's determinants and coping strategies. *Indian Journal of Psychiatry*, *66*(Suppl 2), S231–S244. https://doi.org/10.4103/indianjpsychiatry.indianjpsychiatry_707_23

Goldin, P. R., & Gross, J. J. (2010). Effects of mindfulness-based stress reduction (MBSR) on emotion regulation in social anxiety disorder. *Emotion*, *10*(1), 83–91. https://doi.org/10.1037/a0018441

Gupta, S. (2023, July 10). *How trauma can affect your window of tolerance*. Verywell Mind. https://www.verywellmind.com/window-of-tolerance-7553021

Hoshaw, C. (2022, March 29). *What is mindfulness? A simple practice for greater wellbeing*. Healthline. https://www.healthline.com/health/mind-body/what-is-mindfulness

Isako, S., & Wong, Y. (2010, April 3). *Reiki and pain: One woman's story*. Reikiinmedicine.org. https://reikiinmedicine.org/healthful-lifestyle/reiki-pain-one-womans-story/

Johns Hopkins Medicine. (2019). *The power of positive thinking*. Johns Hopkins Medicine Health Library.

https://www.hopkinsmedicine.org/health/wellness-and-prevention/the-power-of-positive-thinking

Johnson, G. (2019). *How can I do the PSYCH-K method to myself?* Quora. https://www.quora.com/How-can-I-do-the-PSYCH-K-method-to-myself

Johnson, J. (2023, February 9). *What is diaphragmatic breathing? Benefits and how-to.* Www.medicalnewstoday.com. https://www.medicalnewstoday.com/articles/diaphragmatic-breathing

König, N., Steber, S., Seebacher, J., von Prittwitz, Q., Bliem, H. R., & Rossi, S. (2019). How therapeutic tapping can alter neural correlates of emotional prosody processing in anxiety. *Brain Sciences, 9*(8). https://doi.org/10.3390/brainsci9080206

Korn, L. E., Logsdon, R. G., Polissar, N. L., Gomez-Beloz, A., Waters, T. M., & Ryser, R. C. (2012). P02.84. A randomized trial of Polarity therapy for stress and pain reduction in American Indian and Alaska Native family dementia caregivers. *National Library of Medicine, 12*(S1). https://doi.org/10.1186/1472-6882-12-s1-p140

Kuhfuß, M., Maldei, T., Hetmanek, A., & Baumann, N. (2021). Somatic experiencing – effectiveness and key factors of a body-oriented trauma therapy: a scoping literature review. *European Journal of Psychotraumatology, 12*(1),

1929023. https://doi.org/10.1080/20008198.2021.1929023

Kylie. (n.d.). *Rob Williams biography and review of PSYCH-K*. A Guide for Life. https://aguideforlife.com/teacher/rob-williams/

Lambert, J., Ouellet, N., & Boucher, D. (2019). The effect of a polarity intervention on the insomnia and anxiety in middle-aged Quebec women]. *Recherche En Soins Infirmiers, N° 136*(1), 43–53. https://doi.org/10.3917/rsi.136.0043

Lebow, H. (2022, September 14). *How does your body remember trauma? Plus 5 ways to heal*. Psych Central. https://psychcentral.com/health/how-your-body-remembers-trauma

Lebow, H. (2023, January 21). *How does your body remember trauma? Plus 5 ways to heal*. Psych Central. https://psychcentral.com/health/how-your-body-remembers-trauma

Levin, J. (2011). Energy healers: Who they are and what they do. *Explore (New York, N.Y.), 7*(1), 13–26. https://doi.org/10.1016/j.explore.2010.10.005

McKy, K. (n.d.). *How does psych-k work? A whole-brain state is created around a belief*. Subconscious Change with Karen McKy. https://subconsciouschange.com/psych-k-workshops-2/how-does-psych-k-work/

McManus, D. (2017). Reiki is better than placebo and has broad potential as a complementary health therapy. *Journal of Evidence-Based Complementary & Alternative Medicine, 22*(4),

1051–1057. https://doi.org/10.1177/2156587217728644

Mind Motion. (2023). Self-Guided EMDR therapy session with spoken instructions. In *YouTube*. https://www.youtube.com/watch?v=Ljss_Ut5pxY

Mock, S. E., & Arai, S. M. (2011). Childhood trauma and chronic illness in adulthood: Mental health and socioeconomic status as explanatory factors and buffers. *Frontiers in Psychology*, *1*(246). https://doi.org/10.3389/fpsyg.2010.00246

Montes, C., & Penzenstadler, B. (2023). Improved wellbeing and resilience via breathwork interventions for computer workers. *Research Gate*. https://doi.org/10.21203/rs.3.rs-3192152/v1

Murray, M., & Nowicki, J. (2020). *Psychoneuroimmunology*. Www.sciencedirect.com. https://www.sciencedirect.com/topics/medicine-and-dentistry/psychoneuroimmunology

Mustian, K. M., Roscoe, J. A., Palesh, O. G., Sprod, L. K., Heckler, C. E., Peppone, L. J., Usuki, K. Y., Ling, M. N., Brasacchio, R. A., & Morrow, G. R. (2011). Polarity therapy for cancer-related fatigue in patients with breast cancer receiving radiation therapy: A randomized controlled pilot study. *Integrative Cancer Therapies*, *10*(1), 27–37. https://doi.org/10.1177/1534735410397044

*Myths and misconceptions about reiki: Debunking common myths - omega hub*. (2024, April 30). Omega Hub. https://omegahub.co.uk/reiki-healing/reiki-myths/

Nardone, R., Sebastianelli, L., & Saltuari, L. (2017). How the brain can rewire itself after an injury: the lesson from hemispherectomy. *Neural Regeneration Research*, *12*(9), 1426. https://doi.org/10.4103/1673-5374.215247

National Cancer Institute. (2011, February 2). *Homeostasis*. Www.cancer.gov; National Cancer institute. https://www.cancer.gov/publications/dictionaries/cancer-terms/def/homeostasis

Nesci, N. (2020, March 4). 5 things everyone needs to know about energy healing. *The Growth & Wellness Therapy Centre*. https://www.growthwellnesstherapy.com/our-blog/5-things-everyone-needs-to-know-about-energy-healing

Newsom, R., & Rehman, A. (2023, March 3). *The connection between diet, exercise, and sleep*. Sleep Foundation.

https://www.sleepfoundation.org/physical-health/diet-exercise-sleep

Oerman, A. (2023, November 7). *I tried energy healing so you don't have to.* Wondermind. https://www.wondermind.com/article/energy-healing/

Origin stories: Reiki. (2020, October 15). *Isbborne.* https://www.isbourne.org/blog/the-origin-of-reiki

Ortner, C. N. M., Briner, E. L., & Marjanovic, Z. (2017). Believing is doing: Emotion regulation beliefs are associated with emotion regulation behavioral choices and subjective well-being. *Europe's Journal of Psychology, 13*(1), 60–74. https://doi.org/10.5964/ejop.v13i1.1248

Pacini, A. (2021, July 25). *How PSYCH-K helped me heal from a 30-year struggle with disordered eating.* Saltstarlight. https://saltstarlight.com/blogs/self-care-sunday-blog-posts/how-psych-k%C2%AE-helped-me-heal-from-a-30-year-struggle-with-food-addiction-and-disordered-eating?srsltid=AfmBOoqQlBmoAY0XqBL4DdtsBd6I3BOlCoPsl0HuZ6lKdc3KZmv0EvPF

Patel, K. (2022, July 26). *Reiki healing for beginners - how to do reiki.* Goop. https://goop.com/wellness/spirituality/reiki-for-beginners/

Patil, S., Deo, A., & Sharanappa Gornale, S. (2024). A systematic review of human biofield image analysis using image processing techniques. *Journal of the Oriental Institute, 72*(1), 87–98. https://www.researchgate.net/publication/377767791_

A_Systematic_Review_of_Human_Biofield_Image_analysis_using_Image_Processing_Techniques

Perry, E. (2024, June 15). Self-Concept: What is it, and can it change? *Betterup.* https://www.betterup.com/blog/self-concept

Persensky, M. (2021, August 29). *What is reiki, and does it really work?* Cleveland Clinic. https://health.clevelandclinic.org/reiki

Pineda, M. (2022, September). How to muscle test yourself for self-healing. *Connect Heal Expand.* https://thespaciousbreath.com/blog/how-to-muscle-test-yourself-for-self-healing

Pistoia, J. (2022, April 18). *What is polarity therapy.* Psych Central. https://psychcentral.com/health/polarity-therapy

*Polyvagal therapy.* (2018). Counseling and Wellness Center of Pittsburgh, Marriage Counseling, Therapy, and Family Counseling in Pittsburgh, Monroeville, Wexford, and South Hills. https://counselingwellnesspgh.com/counseling/polyvagal-therapy/

Price, R. B., & Duman, R. (2019). Neuroplasticity in cognitive and psychological mechanisms of depression: An integrative model. *Molecular Psychiatry*, *25*(3). https://doi.org/10.1038/s41380-019-0615-x

*Romans 12:2 in-context*. (n.d.). Bible Study Tools. https://www.biblestudytools.com/romans/12-2.html

Russell, J. (2021, March 12). The science of holotropic breathwork in healing trauma. *Jazmine Russell*. https://www.jazminerussell.com/blog/the-science-of-holotropic-breathwork-in-healing-trauma

Schulz, R. (2023, October 17). What to expect before, during, and after an EFT session. *Rochelle Schulz EFT/Tapping*. https://www.rochelleschulz.com/blog-1/what-to-expect-before-during-and-after-an-eft-session

SenGupta, D. (2020, April 30). *4 techniques to ground, heal, & balance your energy levels*. Mindbodygreen. https://www.mindbodygreen.com/articles/how-to-ground-heal-balance-your-energy-levels

*The science of heartmath*. (2017, September 11). HeartMath. https://www.heartmath.com/science/

Shah, P. (2020, October 6). *I'm a master reiki teacher, and here's how I practice self-healing on a regular basis*. Well+Good. https://www.wellandgood.com/reiki-self-healing/

Showers, C. J., Ditzfeld, C. P., & Zeigler-Hill, V. (2014). Self-Concept structure and the quality of self-knowledge.

*Journal of Personality*, *83*(5), 535–551. https://doi.org/10.1111/jopy.12130

Smith, P. (2019, June 19). *The biology of belief – Bruce Lipton*. Mind Spirit Body. https://mindspiritbody.com.au/the-biology-of-belief-full-lecture-bruce-lipton/

Sones, B., & Sones, R. (2018, October 9). *Strange but true: 95 percent of brain activity is unconscious*. The Oklahoman. https://www.oklahoman.com/story/lifestyle/2018/10/09/strange-but-true-95-percent-of-brain-activity-is-unconscious/60496296007/

Stapleton, P., Crighton, G., Sabot, D., & O'Neill, H. M. (2020). Reexamining the effect of emotional freedom techniques on stress biochemistry: A randomized controlled trial. *Psychological Trauma: Theory, Research, Practice, and Policy*, *12*(8). https://doi.org/10.1037/tra0000563

Valera, S. (2023, March 8). *Best mood tracker apps*. Verywell Mind. https://www.verywellmind.com/best-mood-tracker-apps-5212922

van der Kolk, B. (1994). The body keeps the score: Memory and the evolving psychobiology of posttraumatic stress.

*Harvard Review of Psychiatry, 1*(5), 253–265. https://doi.org/10.3109/10673229409017088

van der Kolk, B. (2014). *The body keeps the score: brain, mind and body in the healing of trauma.* Penguin Books.

Vorvick, L. (2023, February 2). *Breathing.* Medlineplus.gov. https://medlineplus.gov/ency/anatomyvideos/000018.htm

WebMD Editorial Contributors. (2023, April 30). *What is box breathing?* WebMD. https://www.webmd.com/balance/what-is-box-breathing

WebMD Editorial Contributors. (2021, October 25). *What is EFT tapping?* WebMD. https://www.webmd.com/balance/what-is-eft-tapping

Welch, A. (2023, July 11). *What is energy healing?* EverydayHealth.com. https://www.everydayhealth.com/integrative-health/energy-healing/guide/

*Welcome to PSYCH-K® and the Evolution of Consciousness | PSYCH-K Centre International.* (n.d.). PSYCH-K Center

International. Retrieved August 1, 2024, from https://psych-k.com/about/

*What is PSYCH-K and how does it work?* (n.d.). The Mindful Coach. https://www.themindfulcoach.com.au/psych-k/

*What is the history of Reiki?* (2014, October 15). Reiki. https://www.reiki.org/faqs/what-history-reiki

*Who developed polarity therapy?* (2014). Polarity Therapy Institute. https://polaritytherapy.com/history

Wilkes, R., & Vartuli, C. (2023, May 29). *History of tapping (including EFT)*. Thriving Now. https://www.thrivingnow.com/history-of-tapping-eft/

Yadav, M. (2022). Diet, sleep and exercise: The keystones of healthy lifestyle for medical students. *Journal of Nepal Medical Association*, *60*(253), 841–843. https://doi.org/10.31729/jnma.7355

Yetman, D. (2020, October 29). *Polarity balancing: Health benefits and how it works*. Healthline; Healthline Media. https://www.healthline.com/health/polarity-balancing

Zaccaro, A., Piarulli, A., Laurino, M., Garbella, E., Menicucci, D., Neri, B., & Gemignani, A. (2018). How breath-control can change your life: A systematic review on psycho-physiological correlates of slow breathing. *Frontiers in Human Neuroscience*, *12*(353), 1–16. https://doi.org/10.3389/fnhum.2018.00353

Zadro, S., & Stapleton, P. (n.d.). Does reiki benefit mental health symptoms above placebo? *Frontiers*, *13*. https://doi.org/doi.org/10.3389/fpsyg.2022.897312

www.ingramcontent.com/pod-product-compliance
Lightning Source LLC
Chambersburg PA
CBHW020535030426
42337CB00013B/855